W9-AXC-329

Baby Boomers
and Hearing Loss

Baby Boomers
and Hearing Loss
A Guide to Prevention
and Care

JOHN M. BURKEY

Rutgers University Press
New Brunswick, New Jersey, and London

Library of Congress Cataloging-in-Publication Data

Burkey, John M., 1959–
    Baby boomers and hearing loss : a guide to prevention and care / John M. Burkey.
        p. cm.
    Includes bibliographical references and index.
    ISBN-13: 978-0-8135-3881-5 (hardcover : alk. paper)
    1. Deafness.   2. Baby boom generation—Health aspects.   3. Older people—Health aspects.   I. Title.
    RF290.B87   2006
    617.8'00846—dc22   2005035515

A British Cataloging-in-Publication record for this book is available from the British Library.

Manufactured in the United States of America

Contents

List of Illustrations   vii

Acknowledgments   ix

Introduction   1

1. What's the Big Deal about Hearing Loss?   5
   How Hearing Loss May Affect You   8
   How Your Hearing Loss May Affect Others   14
   Conclusion   17

2. Baby Boomers and Hearing Loss   18
   Who Are These Baby Boomers?   18
   Special Concerns for Baby Boomers   21
   Some Final Words about Baby Boomers
      and Hearing Loss   27

3. How the Ear Works   28
   Understanding the Ear   29
   Understanding the Types of Hearing Loss   34
   Understanding a Hearing Test   37

4. Causes and Treatments for Hearing Loss   47
   Preventable Hearing Loss   47
   Treatable Hearing Loss   53
   Surmountable Hearing Loss   62

5. Hearing Aid Basics   65
   Hearing Aid Styles   65
   Hearing Aid Circuits   72

Hearing Aid Options   75

Other Hearing Aid Basics   79

6. Satisfaction and Dissatisfaction with
   Hearing Aids   84

   Hearing Aid Benefits   87

   Hearing Aid Satisfaction   89

   Concluding Remarks about Hearing Aid
      Satisfaction   95

7. Non–Hearing Aid Solutions   96

   Having a Plan   97

   Having the Tools   102

8. New and Future Options   110

   Prevention   110

   Surgery   113

   Hearing Aids   118

   A Cure   121

   Getting More Information   123

9. The Issues That Remain   125

   Hearing Aids Revisited   125

   About Insurance   133

   Hearing Research   134

   Connecting the Dots   135

   Resources   139

   References   151

   Index   167

Illustrations

Figure 3.1. The human ear   30

Figure 3.2. The middle ear   31

Figure 3.3. Audiogram showing normal hearing   40

Figure 3.4. Audiogram showing a conductive hearing loss   44

Figure 3.5. Audiogram showing a sensorineural hearing loss   45

Figure 3.6. Audiogram showing a mixed hearing loss   45

Figure 5.1. Sizes and landmarks of in-the-ear hearing aids   66

Figure 5.2. Landmarks of a behind-the-ear hearing aid
with earmold   66

Figure 8.1. Surgically implanted portion of a cochlear
implant   113

Figure 8.2. Externally worn cochlear implant sound
processor   114

Figure 8.3. Parts of the BAHA system   116

Figure 8.4. BAHA sound transmission for single-sided
deafness   117

Acknowledgments

I thank Beth Kressel, editorial assistant at Rutgers University Press, for her many insightful comments and suggestions during the preparation of this book. I also thank Audra Wolfe, Ph.D., science editor, and Kathryn Gohl, copyeditor. *Baby Boomers and Hearing Loss* is my second book with Rutgers. It has been my privilege to twice benefit from the favorable publishing environment they provide.

I additionally thank the physicians, audiologists, nurses, and support staff at the Lippy Group for Ear, Nose, and Throat for their encouragement throughout this project. Finally, I thank my wife, Karen, for her love and understanding during the writing and publication process.

Introduction

A decrease in hearing as we age is nothing new. But hearing loss has never met such a fearsome opponent as the typical baby boomer who works hard on the job with no immediate plans for retirement, smashes overheads on the tennis court after work, attends rock concerts on Saturday evenings, shops for the latest cellular phone, and plans to upgrade from VHS tape to TiVo any day now. Of course, hearing is essential for all of these activities.

If we are concerned about maintaining a youthful quality of life, keeping our senses sharp, particularly our hearing, is key. This book explains how to determine whether you are hearing as well as you should. It explains the medical, surgical, and technological interventions that are available now to correct or compensate for hearing loss. And if your sense of sound is still 100 percent, the book suggests how to keep it that way. Because many forms of hearing loss cannot be reversed, recognizing potential causes and avoiding them is the best medicine. Furthermore, the quality, scope, and availability of future auditory care will be the direct result of decisions made today. You may wish to support or promote hearing-related programs or legislation, explained in later chapters, from which you could benefit.

Hearing well now is no guarantee of hearing well in the future, especially because the likelihood of hearing loss increases with age. Compared with previous generations, baby boomers face an increased risk of hearing loss and a greater need to preserve their sense of sound.

First, baby boomers are expected to live longer than previous generations and the likelihood of hearing loss is directly related to aging. In 1900, when the average life expectancy was forty-seven years, age related hearing loss was not a serious problem. But baby boomers, that is, those born between 1946 and 1964, have an average life expectancy of seventy years (Arias et al. 2003). The 10 percent incidence of hearing loss reported for the general population (National Institute on Deafness and Other Communication Disorders, 1989) is bad enough, but people over the age of seventy are more than three times as likely to be hard of hearing. Those who live beyond the age of eighty-five have five times the incidence or a one in two chance of suffering hearing loss (Desai et al. 2001). Obviously, hearing loss should be a concern for baby boomers.

Political realities also make hearing important for baby boomers. Simply reaching sixty-five years of age is no longer a guarantee of retirement. The eligibility age for Social Security is already increasing. The baby bust that followed the baby boom leaves too few people paying taxes to support their elders. Although a person's continued ability to hear is likely to have a direct impact on his or her employability, baby boomers may not have the option, as their parents or grandparents did, to leave the workplace in their sixties.

Continued hearing will also be a lifestyle issue. Baby boomers are not likely to quietly accept limitations or a reduced quality of life. Whether it is music, fashion, art, or politics, baby boomers have demonstrated more than a slight disregard for limits, and it is unlikely that their approach to hearing loss will be any different. More positively, baby boomers have hearing care options not available to their parents that will help them continue to experience a sound-rich life.

As a clinical audiologist and director of audiology at a busy ear, nose, and throat clinic, I have had the privilege of working closely with a variety of healthcare professionals, including physicians, surgeons, medical researchers, residents, equipment manufacturers, audiologists, hearing instrument specialists, speech pathologists, nurses, nurse practitioners, university professors, deaf educators, and insurance specialists. This has given me a multidisciplinary perspective, which I draw on throughout this volume.

Although this book was written specifically for those born right after World War II, much of the information is relevant for other generations, including teens or elders.

The first chapter deals with perhaps the most important issue in this book—why we should worry about hearing loss. Because hearing is such an integral part of so much that we do, even a mild hearing loss can significantly impact our relationships, work, leisure, safety, and security. Social science studies and personal narratives show how hearing loss (ours or someone else's) can be detrimental. Chapter 2 explores the cultural and financial factors that make it crucial for us to hear well.

A basic grasp of the anatomy and function of a normal ear is useful to appreciate what can go wrong. So, to, is an understanding of what constitutes normal hearing and how it is measured. Chapter 3 details the different parts of the ear and their functions in addition to describing a typical audiogram or hearing test and ways to interpret the results. The nuts and bolts provided in chapter three are necessary to understand many ear diseases and their resultant hearing losses. These basics are also essential for evaluating potential medical treatments or surgery.

Chapter 4 focuses on the causes of hearing loss, and possible interventions, including medication or surgery. On occasion, hearing loss may indicate a larger medical problem. I have included a list of "red flag" symptoms to help patients recognize when there may be more to worry about.

Hearing aids are typically the best alternative to compensate for a hearing loss that is not medically correctable. Chapter 5 gives you an overview of this technology including sizing, circuitry (analog versus digital), adjustability, microphone types, telephone compatibility, and the latest advances in the field. Selecting an appropriate hearing aid is not a matter of buying the "latest" or "best" model, but of finding the hearing aid best suited to a person's loss and current lifestyle.

Although hearing aids enhance the hearing of most users, fewer than one in four people who need them use them (Kochkin 2001). Chapter 6 explores the myths that lead people to resist trying the technology. Then, on the basis of scientific studies and user surveys, I explain the pros and cons of hearing aids.

Chapter 7 suggests ways to improve your listening environment. Perhaps this means switching from a traditional to an amplified telephone or sitting closer to the person you are speaking to. Perhaps this means using assistive listening devices above and beyond traditional hearing aids. This chapter is especially valuable for those seeking to improve specific listening situations but who generally have few hearing problems.

Chapter 8 focuses on recent advances in hearing healthcare, including cochlear implants, and potential future breakthroughs. Since the vast majority of hearing loss results from nerve damage that is not currently medically correctable, a breakthrough in the regeneration of these nerves would dramatically improve the quality of life for many.

New technology aside, the final chapter is about taking control. Previous generations did not take advantage of medical and technological options and consequently suffered the effects of their hearing loss. In order to maintain an active lifestyle, baby boomers will need to do better than their parents to shape the options for the future. Petitioning employers to provide hearing care as an insurance benefit and supporting hearing research are just two options.

Finally, the appendix contains a list of resources, including information about magazines, books, medical and audiology associations, self-help groups, newsgroups, and websites.

Although a variety of hearing care issues are discussed throughout this book, the information should not be considered as medical advice nor used in place of appropriate medical care. When describing specific cases, I use pseudonym to protect the patients' confidentiality.

1 What's the Big Deal about Hearing Loss?

When Kathie first came to my office, she was crying as she described her frustration over the hearing loss that had been worsening over a quarter of a century. There was no obvious cause for her hearing loss, although heredity may have played a role since several family members had a similar problem. She also reported ringing in her ears and had worn hearing aids to compensate for her hearing loss and to mask the ringing. She recounted how as her hearing worsened she experienced increasing difficulty understanding people in more and more situations. The aids helped tremendously, but she was still struggling. She could generally understand her husband Sam when they were conversing in quiet settings, but she often misheard him in louder situations. This was placing increasing limits on their social life. Work was an even bigger problem. Kathie and Sam owned and operated a funeral home. They both agreed that the day-to-day goings-on there were emotional enough without misunderstanding the request of a client or responding inappropriately to the bereaved. They had taken special care to decorate with carpeting and other sound-absorbing materials that would limit reverberation. This helped but did not solve the problem. Kathie felt she had received good hearing healthcare where she lived but still wanted another opinion to see what else might be done. Both Kathie and Sam considered the hearing loss such a problem that they drove seven hours to our clinic for a second opinion.

Kathie's situation is not uncommon. Two weeks after meeting her, I counseled a man in a similar situation. He had been trying to help out at a local funeral home since losing his factory job. He was equally frustrated and more than a little bit embarrassed about some of his misunderstandings at his new workplace.

As the stories of Kathie and others show, hearing loss affects everything from relationships to social activities, work, mood, and self-image. A reduced quality of life is the by-product of hearing loss. Beyond anecdotal evidence, surveys and research confirm the demoralizing effects of hearing loss.

Although quality of life is hard to assess because it is so subjective, exploring this concept is important for determining the extent to which poor hearing is affecting a person's life. In an analysis of seventy-five articles on the subject, Gill and Feinstein (1994) concluded that quality of life is a multifaceted personal perception that must be measured from an individual's point of view. The findings did not rule out the use of standardized measures but stressed that these must be supplemented with personal insights.

Quality of life can also be confusing because it is often used interchangeably as a subjective measure of status and as an objective measure of function. This confusion is true even in the scientific literature. A subjective quality-of-life estimate might be achieved by asking someone How do you feel? This approach is much different than the objective measure of a person's blood pressure or pulse rate. The quality-of-life discussions presented in this chapter are primarily about individual perceptions.

Quality of life can additionally be viewed within a global or specific context. A global quality-of-life measure is multidimensional. It looks at a large number of factors that may affect a person's quality of life and averages together their impact. Although this provides a nice "big picture" perspective, it can hide specific problems that a person may consider significant. You might rate your overall quality of life as excellent if you have no limitations except those resulting from a hearing loss. This favorable perception would likely remain even if the hearing loss caused significant limitations. In reality, poor hearing may be causing problems in many life situations, thus leading to a significant reduction in quality of life. For example, you may have excellent ground stokes in tennis, but if you can't hear your opponent call the ball in or out, you'll be ill prepared for the return shot. Similarly, you may be skilled at cards but play poorly due to mishearing the bids. The invitation to either of these activities may be missed if difficulty hearing makes you avoid using the phone. In what specific ways are you being affected by your hearing loss?

Asking how hearing loss affects a person will be of little value if the hearing loss is unrecognized or denied. This does not mean that personal perceptions will be unrevealing. Because a person may be able to describe problems without understanding their causes, we can ask what situations or activities the person feels he or she struggles with. Are there activates that used to be enjoyable but now are not? Maybe a former movie buff finds theaters intolerable, preferring the more intimate viewing of a DVD at home; could this person really be choosing to stay home because it's more conducive to hearing the dialogue? Once the "what" is identified, it then becomes possible to focus on the "why." It can be quite telling when a hearing loss is unsuspected or denied, yet every perceived struggle or limitation is related to hearing.

Interestingly, a person's age group can also affect the perceived impact of hearing loss. In a study of over three thousand middle-aged and older adults, researchers (Wiley et al. 2000) found that although older individuals were more likely to have a hearing loss, they were less likely to report it as a handicap. The possible reasons for this are many. Two of the more obvious ones are activity level and expectations. It should not be surprising that hearing loss is perceived as less of a problem for an older individual who is retired and not very socially active than for a working baby boomer who is socially active. Activity level alone, however, cannot explain this trend since many people remain very active well into old age.

Expectation based on generational differences also plays a role in the perceived impact of hearing loss. Older individuals who struggled or sacrificed during the Great Depression and World War II may expect less from life than baby boomers, who have had more and sacrificed less. Health-related expectations are also likely to be different between age groups. A forty-five-year-old usually expects good health without any limitations, while a seventy-five-year-old may expect a few age-related health problems. This tendency of older individuals to make more global assessments may mask the true impact of hearing loss.

How Hearing Loss May Affect You

Hearing loss does not occur in isolation. It is not some hypothetical construct manifested on the notepads of medical professionals or invented by hearing aid manufacturers. It is a chronic condition with real-life consequences, some more severe than others. The effects are seen on objective tests of function, subjective quality-of-life measures, and individual reports. The areas most affected are discussed here. You may find some to be all too familiar.

Social Functioning

Tina is one of the youngest of the baby boomers. Despite her age, which places her at lower risk of hearing loss compared with other baby boomers, she had been experiencing a progressive hearing loss in both ears for at least six years. She had no history of noise exposure or other controllable environmental factor that might have caused the loss. Her father had a long-standing hearing problem that was especially frustrating for him socially. She wanted something different for herself.

Tina reported constantly having to ask people to repeat themselves. She stated that people feel she is ignoring them because she does not answer. The hearing loss was affecting social interactions, time spent with her husband, and her supervisory position at work. She was especially unnerved that she could not hear when a person would come up behind her.

The one area in which there is no disagreement about hearing loss affecting quality of life is in the realm of social functioning. Because spoken communication is such an integral and pervasive part of our society, anything that reduces a person's ability to understand what is said is bound to be limiting. A 1990 study of male veterans (Mulrow et al.) found that hearing loss was associated with significant social and communicative dysfunction. Most persuasive to the argument was that two-thirds of the veterans perceived their dysfunction as a severe handicap, even though testing showed their hearing losses to be in only the mild or moderate range. Mulrow and colleagues concluded that there was no doubt that hearing loss can negatively affect quality of life, even when the hearing loss is mild.

A larger and more recent investigation returned similar results (Dalton et al. 2003) in which the researchers found that 59 percent of people with a mild hearing loss and 80 percent of those with more severe losses reported significant communication difficulties. The amount of communication difficulty reported was directly related to the severity of the loss. The study also highlighted the fact that hearing loss is frequently an unrecognized and underreported disorder. Of those who reported significant communication difficulties, only 22 percent of people with a mild hearing loss and 56 percent with a more severe loss reported a hearing handicap.

Loneliness and Isolation

The communication difficulties imposed by hearing loss can produce a sense of loneliness and isolation. To document this relationship, a group of researchers administered a loneliness questionnaire to over three thousand people with hearing loss (Kramer et al. 2002). The results from the questionnaire showed a clear relationship between hearing loss and loneliness. The researchers also looked at the issue of loneliness and isolation in a more objective manner. Rather than asking subjects how lonely they felt, the researchers measured how isolated they had become. They accomplished this by counting the number of people in an individual's social network and the number of different types of social groups with which a person interacts. Did a person maintain an important and regular relationship with friends, neighbors, children, co-workers, organizations, and so forth, or was their only contact with the immediate family? They found that the social network of people with hearing loss was significantly smaller than that of their normal hearing peers. The hearing impaired were indeed more isolated.

Reduced Independence

Reduced independence can be another consequence of hearing loss. Although hearing loss does not limit physical mobility, it may limit a person's ability to function alone. Events can take unexpected turns when there is no one to repeat or interpret what was misheard or unheard. A person may be hesitant to deal with banking, investing, and legal matters if he or she does not have confidence in what is heard.

Following a doctor's instructions is difficult if the instructions are not understood. Even a haircut or styling can go wrong if a clarification about cut or color is misunderstood. Situations such as these make a person wary of acting autonomously. The self-limiting of activities that can result from this reduction in confidence can be as detrimental to a person's independence as what may be misheard.

We may think a hearing loss would have to be awfully bad before it could limit a person's independence. This is not, unfortunately, the case. An investigation in the *Journal of Rehabilitation Research and Development*, which looked at just this issue (Scherer and Frisina 1998), found that even a marginal hearing loss caused people to report less satisfaction with their independence than was reported by people with normal hearing.

Safety and security concerns can also act to limit independence. A person may not feel comfortable living alone if fire, smoke, or burglar alarms are inaudible. Not being able to hear surrounding sounds may make walking through a park or down a neighborhood sidewalk appear risky. Not being able to hear or localize road sounds may make a person less likely to drive. These are only a few of the safety and security concerns that can curb a hearing-impaired person's independence.

Tiredness

Baby boomers are often characterized by their tremendous enthusiasm and energy, but difficulty hearing can inhibit this joie de vivre. People with a known hearing loss often report that they understand better when they concentrate on what is said. People in denial of a hearing loss frequently say they only misunderstand when they are not paying attention. Each group recognizes that they understand better when they focus. In actuality they are filling in missing parts of words and missing words in sentences. Also, most languages are fairly redundant in how they convey what is said. Take for example the sentence "I am going to the grocery store to buy some chocolate chip cookies." It would be relatively easy to correctly fill in a missed word or two. Missed letters can also be deciphered from the context of the sentence. They can additionally be inferred from the way one spoken sound influences another. Listen to the letter *a* when saying *car* and *cap.* The different mouth positions required to say the letters *r* and *p* make the *a* sound different. If the final letter were missed, the sound of the *a* could be used to narrow down the possibilities for this last letter.

Although a hearing-impaired person can understand better by focusing on and thinking about what is said, this is not accomplished without effort. Trying to decipher what is not heard can be hard work. The more that is missed, the harder it is. Listening with noise in the background or while multiple people are talking is especially difficult because there is more to sort out. It is also difficult to understand people who talk fast. There may be insufficient time to figure out what might have been missed. Listening situations that may be effortless for a person with normal hearing can be exhausting for a person with hearing loss. Rather than being so tired at the end of the day, some individuals will not make the effort to hear and understand. Lethargy is in fact an often-reported consequence of hearing loss (Heine and Browning 2002).

Depression

Considering the many ways a hearing loss can negatively affect an individual, we should not be surprised that depression might result. Although not everyone who suffers hearing loss will develop depression, hearing loss definitely increases the likelihood. Heine and Browning (2002) noted that depression was an often-reported consequence of hearing loss. A separate study of age-related hearing difficulties found that 14 percent of the subjects experienced a depressed mood. Their negative mood was attributed to declining hearing (Vesterager et al. 1988).

It is not necessary that a person be aware of a hearing loss to suffer depression as a result. Reduced enjoyment in social situations, feelings of isolation, loneliness, reduced confidence, anxiety, stress, and tiredness can all lead to depression. Some people seek treatment for their state of mind only to find that the solution is treatment for their hearing loss.

Reduced Cognitive Functioning

Hearing loss has also been associated with reduced cognitive abilities. A review of studies examining the negative consequences of hearing loss (Arlinger 2003) found that most investigations discovered a correlation between hearing loss and reduced cognitive function. The significance of this correlation, however, was not always clear. The design of many studies did not allow the investigators to differentiate whether the reduced cognitive abilities occurred along with the hearing loss or because of the hearing loss. They could not rule out the possibility that both problems were caused by a general age-related degeneration or some other factor. A couple of the better-designed studies that were reviewed indicated that hearing loss caused cognitive decline. More research will likely be needed before we can definitively point toward hearing loss as a contributing factor to cognitive decline, but the evidence is leaning in that direction.

Employment

There are laws that prevent discrimination in the hiring of hearing-impaired workers. Laws also exist requiring employers to make reasonable accommodations for existing employees who have or who develop hearing loss. These might include providing an employee with an amplified telephone, conducting business through e-mail rather than by phone, or moving an employee to a position that does not require excellent hearing. Changes such as these can help a person to remain gainfully employed and be an asset to an employer.

At the beginning of this chapter, I recounted how Kathie's hearing difficulties caused her to struggle with the duties in her funeral home business. Misunderstandings were common. Special requests went unheard. She was upset and frustrated because this sometimes made her appear insensitive or incompetent. Her story illustrated only a few of the work-related difficulties that can be caused by hearing loss.

An employee may have on-going problems with hearing in the workplace for many reasons: noise, workplace acoustics, necessary listening demands, or the severity of the hearing loss. Consequently, a person with hearing loss may have to work harder to perform a specific job than a worker with normal hearing. Struggling with a hearing loss may also make a job more stressful. Although special accommodations and guarantees against discrimination are helpful in the workplace, they do not entirely negate the consequences of hearing loss.

Being able to perform the job is only one workplace issue. Equally important is enjoying the job. Unfortunately, hearing loss also causes trouble here. A large part of what makes working enjoyable is the social interaction between co-workers, workers and customers, clients, or patients. Waitresses do not usually derive enjoyment from setting down and picking up plates. They enjoy the social interaction with their customers. Nurses enjoy caring for and getting to know their patients. We discuss sports, television, music, children, politics, and more with the people we see at work. These discussions can be the most pleasurable part of the workday. The negative effects of hearing loss on social functioning have already been discussed. These issues clearly apply in the workplace.

Not surprisingly, people with hearing loss are less likely to be employed full time than are those with normal hearing (Dalton et al. 2003). Although this finding is relational rather than causal, it raises economic in addition to quality-of-life concerns.

All of the Above

The consequences of hearing loss are usually far-reaching, as reported in 2000 by the National Council on Aging. The council reported that people with untreated hearing loss were more likely to suffer sadness, depression, worry, anxiety, paranoia, insecurity, emotional turmoil, and reduced social activity compared with their peers.

Kramer and colleagues (2002) also found the effects of hearing loss to be wide ranging. They reported that people with hearing loss were more likely to experience depression, loneliness, and feelings of being externally controlled or controlled by the situation. The hearing impaired additionally had a smaller social network and a lower expectation that they could achieve their goals. These psychosocial variables were examined for a variety of chronic diseases (cancer, lung disease, diabetes, stroke, and so forth) in addition to hearing loss. Although each of these diseases was found to have negative psychosocial consequences, only hearing loss was found to adversely affect outcomes on all of the psychosocial measures examined. The conclusion of this study was that hearing loss clearly affects quality of life.

How Your Hearing Loss May Affect Others

Burt, a fifty-three-year-old autoworker, was brought to our office by his wife, Barb, and teenage daughter Terri. He reported a long history of noise exposure, including military service, recreational shooting, the use of power tools, tractors, and motorcycles, loud music, and industrial noise. He usually did not use ear protection when engaging in noisy activities. Although he acknowledged some difficulty hearing if a person mumbled or talked quietly, he said he didn't think his hearing was a problem.

His wife and daughter felt differently. They were tired of having to repeat themselves. Both complained of being lectured on how to speak clearly. Burt blamed anything that he misheard on the speaker. Barb could not enjoy television or a movie because she missed what was said while repeating things to her husband. The television was often so loud that Terri could not concentrate on her homework, regardless of where she went in the house. Barb felt awkward having to explain why Burt was avoiding church gatherings and other social activities. Terri didn't like it when her friends asked "What's wrong with your dad?" Although the hearing loss wasn't theirs, it was Barb and Terri who wanted help.

Imagine an evening of television watching with Burt and Barb. Both sit down to watch the forensic crime show *CSI*. Burt turns the volume as high as it can go and still can't make out all of the words. His teenage daughter, finishing up some calculus homework, yells down the stairs to turn the volume down. The show's investigators have analyzed all of the evidence and are about to explain who committed the murder and why it was done. Just then, Burt asks Barb what one of the characters had said. As she explains, both of them miss the most important part of the show. Their daughter storms out of the house, demanding peace and quiet for her studies. Everyone is frustrated.

We can see that a person with hearing loss is not the only one affected by the handicap. It touches spouses, children, friends, coworkers, acquaintances, and even bystanders. Ignoring a hearing loss affects everyone. Research has shown it to have a negative impact on spouses, family, friends, and others. Issues frequently raised by

significant others of the hearing impaired included annoyance over their loved one's dependence, irritation, and feelings of frustration all around. Frustration over having to repeat oneself and numerous other communication problems were also mentioned (Stephens et al. 1995; Brooks et al. 2001). Several of these issues arise during the most mundane activities such as television watching.

Communication Difficulties

No one is surprised if a person with hearing loss complains about communication difficulties. What surprises many is that this same hearing loss can cause problems for others. The reason for this confusion is that at the mention of communication problems, most people think about difficulty understanding. They do not think about difficulty being understood. Recall Barb having to repeat herself while explaining some missed dialogue to Burt.

One of the biggest challenges and frustrations for significant others of a person with hearing loss is trying to be understood. Repetition may always seem necessary. Extra effort has to be made to talk louder or directly to the hearing-impaired person. All of this can also be a frustration for casual acquaintances. The added effort to be understood and frustration at being misunderstood can make an encounter less enjoyable and possibly less likely to happen in the future. A decision by friends or acquaintances to spend less time may not be made at a conscious level. They simply spend more time doing what they enjoy and less time doing what they do not. This is one contributing factor explaining why hearing-impaired persons often feel isolated and have a smaller social network.

Responsibility and Dependency

Family or friends are often surprised and frustrated to find that the problems resulting from a hearing-impaired person's hearing difficulties have become their responsibility. More is involved than just repeating. Family or friends may be expected to accompany the hearing-impaired person during social situations or on simple outings to the grocery or convenience store. Someone with hearing loss may expect help when dealing with financial, legal, or tax specialists. Even ordering pizza may become someone else's responsibility if hearing on the phone is difficult. So common is the expectation to hear in everyday life that there are countless little things a hearing-impaired person could use help with. The cumulative effect of these needs can become an unwanted barrage to family and friends.

Imposed Limitations

Previously I discussed how those with hearing loss often withdraw from social activities. Often overlooked is how this withdrawal can have a negative impact on significant others. Because married people engage in many activities as a couple, any limitation on one can become a limitation for both. If hearing loss prevents a person from enjoying a concert, it may result in both that person and his spouse forgoing concerts. If a person avoids church gatherings, class reunions, movies, restaurants, and the like because of difficulty hearing, then she may be limiting these activities for her spouse. In turn, a spouse may be choosing to limit activities to those that do not cause difficulty to the hearing-impaired partner. In either case, both parties are affected.

Stress

Coping with the hearing loss of a partner can be stressful. This is true even when a hearing-impaired person is doing the best he or she can and their spouse is understanding and supportive. It is worse when a hearing loss is unrecognized or denied and the spouse is viewed as one of the causes of communication difficulties. If a person's hearing is not the perceived problem, then it must be the way a spouse speaks. No better is when a hearing loss is recognized but a person makes no effort to deal with it. Burt's daughter felt burdened when her dad turned the television volume up and she could not focus on her homework. In addition, spouses become responsible for what goes unheard and can even become resentful that this burden may be unnecessary.

Numerous stories have appeared in the media identifying stress as the cause for physical and psychological ills. There is little scientific argument that stress can have negative consequences. This relationship remains true when the stress is caused by the hearing loss of another. A long-term study examining the impact of hearing loss found that spousal hearing loss increased the likelihood of subsequent poorer physical, psychological, and social health in partners (Wallhagan et al. 2004).

Conclusion

One of my most touching cases involved a concerned business owner and her employee. Linda explained that she was the owner of a retail and wholesale auto parts business and that Patty had worked many years as her receptionist, cashier, and phone secretary. She noticed that Patty was having more and more trouble understanding customers on the phone and in person. Patty had also gotten several customer orders wrong. Linda wanted to keep her as an employee but felt she could not afford to let Patty remain in her present position unless something were to change. Moving Patty to a position that did not require good hearing might have been an option if there were an opening, but there was not. Furthermore, she did not want to spend the time and money to find and train a replacement. Linda said that although the company's health insurance did not cover ear or hearing evaluations, she would pay for an examination herself to see if Patty could be helped.

The information presented in this chapter clearly shows that hearing loss is a significant problem. It can reduce a person's quality of life as well as the quality of life of those around an individual. But as we see in later chapters, Patty and the other patients described were able to mitigate their disability in a variety of ways.

Forthcoming chapters discuss the medical and technological interventions that can prevent hearing loss from causing a reduction in quality of life. Outcomes for the personal stories described here are discussed in later chapters as the appropriate intervention for each is introduced. Before delving into the causes and solutions for hearing loss, however, we first examine why hearing loss presents a special problem for baby boomers.

2   Baby Boomers and Hearing Loss

The baby boom generation does not have an exclusive claim to the problem of hearing loss. Previous generations have suffered, and hearing loss will likely be a problem for future generations. There are, however, a number of factors that combine to make hearing loss especially problematic for baby boomers. To understand how this handicap will impact baby boomers, we start with a brief look at this generation.

Who Are These Baby Boomers?

You who are baby boomers know who you are. Beyond this, it is as difficult to categorize this generation as it is to choose a high-profile figure who might be representative of the generation. Baby boomers include the political opposites of Bill Clinton and George W. Bush, and the genius and entrepreneurial spirit of Bill Gates, who molded Microsoft into the software giant it is today. On the other hand, boomers include Terry Nichols and Timothy McVeigh, who were convicted of the Oklahoma City bombing. We might look to James Taylor and Jon Mellencamp as representative of the musical tastes of this generation. Yet how can we overlook the country music of Garth Brooks, the rock of Jon Bon Jovi, the pop of Michael Jackson, the disco of Donna Summer, the piano stylings of Jim Brickman, and numerous other genres embraced by baby boomers.

Just as there are many baby boomer icons, this group defies a single categorization. A number of past attempts are shown in box 2.1. None adequately describes the baby boom generation.

Years ago it was very common to label baby boomers as the Woodstock or antiwar generation. Peace, love, and rock and roll was the mantra of the day. At the same time, a cold war and an arms race were occurring. Living with the specter of nuclear annihilation was

---

Box 2.1. Categorizations and nicknames for the baby boom generation

Woodstock/hippie generation	Rock and roll generation
Vietnam/antiwar generation	Dr. Spock generation
Cold war generation	Space race generation
Television generation	Pepsi generation
Me generation	Education generation
Modern/young generation	Credit card generation
A-bomb generation	New Age generation

---

abhorrent yet at the same time commonplace and accepted. Individual baby boomers espoused and continue to support a wide range of views from pacifism to militarism.

Baby boomers have been characterized in terms of the science and technology they have enjoyed. In an age in which people could travel into space, beyond the bounds of earth's atmosphere, and to the moon, anything seemed possible. At the same time, other baby boomers embraced mysticism, spirituality, altered states of consciousness, and less scientific views. Many avoided the technological and artificial in favor of the more natural.

Baby boomers were certainly the first television generation. This medium reached into the living rooms of nearly all boomers, whose viewing may have included such staid programming as *Father Knows Best* or the more comedic *Rowan and Martin's Laugh-In*. Advertisers embraced television and made every possible use of this medium to capture the baby boomer as consumer. Naming them the Pepsi generation turned out to be one ingenious marketing coup. Fast-food restaurants, auto companies, beer distributors, and everyone else who had a product to sell also got in on the act. Yet with the billions spent on advertising, there is really no one product that defines the generation. Interestingly, all of this advertising may have been instrumental in earning baby boomers the title of the "me" generation by instilling an expectation of immediate gratification. Without doubt, the emergence of credit cards (which were also advertised on television) additionally played a role.

In the 1980 book *Great Expectations: America and the Baby Boom Generation,* Landon Jones depicted the baby boomers in all their complexity. He examined the factors that led to the baby boom, how these children were viewed by their parents and by society, and what the boomers said and believed about themselves. He also looked at the fads and trends they spawned, their music, politics, protests, and entrance into the workforce. Midlife and beyond were predicted with surprising accuracy. He recognized that it was next to impossible to view baby boomers outside the context of the Vietnam War, the cold war, politics, civil rights, music, drugs, the sexual revolution, women's liberation, and other events of their time. These turbulent times shaped baby boomers into a very diverse generation. What he ultimately concluded, however, was that it was not politics and culture but the overwhelming size of the baby boom generation that most shaped and defined them.

The generally accepted and most unambiguous definition of a baby boomer is a person born in the years between 1946 and 1964, when the birthrate truly boomed. The number of births in the United States during in the 1930s and early 1940s averaged 2.5 to 3 million per year. During the baby boom years of 1946 to 1964, births jumped to an average 4 million per year. By 1965 the number of children born dropped below 4 million, and the yearly birthrate did not again reach this number until nearly twenty-five years later. By the early 1970s the yearly birthrate had dropped back to nearly 3 million (Martin et al. 2002). This period was termed the baby bust. Before this downturn occurred, however, 76 million baby boomers had been born (Vital and Health Statistics 1964; Martin et al. 2002). Although there was also a baby boom in Canada, Australia, and a few other countries that coincided with the baby boom in the United States, the discussions here focus on the U.S. boomers.

Jones (1980) described the baby boom generation as being the "pig in the python" of the U.S. population. Whether as youngsters, middle-agers, or older, they would disrupt everything with their passage. The generation's size sometimes served as its benefactor; at other times, the reverse. Baby boomer whims became fads. Their fads became trends, and these trends became the societal norm. A smaller generation would have conformed. Instead it was often society that conformed to the baby boomers. Society was unprepared for such an unwieldy group. Their numbers outpaced the construction of nurseries, classrooms, and housing. Hospital birthing centers were overrun. Classroom sizes soared. Housing shortages occurred as baby boomers left home. Entering the workforce was also traumatic. Unemployment rose as millions of boomers sought entry-level jobs that did not exist. Entry-level pay followed the laws of supply and demand and stagnated. Although these disruptions resolved themselves with time, there have been—and will be—others to follow. Jones made clear in his book that as long as the pig is in the python, there are more disruptions to come.

All of these factors that helped define the baby boom generation in youth and middle age, including the diversity of their cultural and political beliefs, their exposure to technology and consumerism, and most importantly, the situations arising as a result of their large numbers, are relevant to how they will cope with the challenges of hearing loss.

Special Concerns for Baby Boomers

As I mentioned in the introduction, the National Institute on Deafness and Other Communication Disorders (1989) has estimated that 28 million Americans or about 10 percent of the U.S. population suffer with hearing loss. Other reports have confirmed this statistic (Ries 1994; Kochkin 1996). Baby boomers, like everyone in the United States, must recognize this baseline statistic before learning how people of their generation may be uniquely affected by the problem.

Noise Exposure and Hearing Loss

Since the industrial revolution, people have coped with hearing loss resulting from noise exposure. Loud sounds can damage the effectiveness of our ears. Knowing this, we might conclude that the many governmental regulations aimed at protecting us from industrial and other noise would give baby boomers a hearing advantage over previous generations. This does not take into account, unfortunately, baby boomers' love of rock and roll, blues, and other amplified music. Many baby boomers have spent a lifetime exposing themselves to potentially damaging levels of music. Surprisingly, the long-term effects of music on hearing can be debated. Research clearly shows that the risk to hearing can be significant if the music is loud enough (Meyer-Bisch 1996). Given most people's average preferred listening level, however, the likelihood of damage may only be slight (Hetu and Fortin 1995). One group of researchers ultimately concluded that the individuals at risk of hearing loss have "maladapted listening patterns," such as the habit of listening to extremely loud music for long periods (Florentine et al. 1998). Although this would not put all baby boomers in jeopardy, it would definitely increase the likelihood of hearing loss for some. Baby boomers who frequent nightclubs or aerobics classes in which the music is often played at damaging levels may also suffer hearing loss at higher rates (Wilson and Herbstain 2003; Bray, Szymanski, and Mills 2004). How many loud places do you routinely frequent after which you experience ear pain, ringing, a plugged sensation, or decreased hearing?

Regardless of how we choose to look at this issue of noise-induced hearing loss (industrial, music, or other), the picture is not promising for baby boomers. An age-adjusted study in Alameda, California, found that the prevalence of hearing loss nearly doubled between 1965 and 1994 (Wallhagen et al. 1997). This trend is not something that any baby boomer should take lightly.

Increasing Age and Hearing Loss

In addition to listening habits, baby boomers must factor in the inevitable decline of hearing in old age. The youngest of the baby boom generation are now entering middle age. The oldest members of this generation are entering their sixth decade of life. Although baby boomers may still count themselves as members of the "young" generation, the math belies this perspective. Baby boomers as a group are approaching old age and the maladies that accompany it.

The incidence and severity of hearing loss increase with age. Just how many people become affected is debatable, depending on how we choose to define hearing loss. The percentage is lowest if we only include those individuals with a more noticeable or handicapping hearing loss. In this case, one-third of the people seventy years of age or older are affected (Desai et al. 2001). If we use this same age group and also include those with a slight but measurable hearing loss, the percentage jumps to 60 (Gratton and Vazquez 2003). Bridging the gap between these extremes is a study in which 46 percent of the older adults of Beaver Dam, Wisconsin (Cruickshanks, Wiley, et al. 1998), were found to suffer hearing loss. The average age of the residents examined was 65.8 years. Baby boomers are headed directly toward these statistics.

Longer Life Expectancy

Not only do baby boomers face the increased prospect of hearing loss as they age, but they will likely live longer with this disability than have previous generations. The average baby boomer has a life expectancy at birth of nearly seventy years, which is four to eight years more than that of the previous generation (Arias 2004). In fact, the expected longevity for baby boomers who are alive today is higher than these statistics suggest because fatalities such as childhood maladies, accidents, and other mishaps have already taken their toll. Statisticians have estimated that men who live to sixty-five years of age can expect to live sixteen years longer and women who live to sixty-five can expect to live nineteen years longer (Desai et al. 2001). These are a lot of years for baby boomers to deal with the prospect of hearing loss.

Retirement

The hordes of baby boomers who are now approaching retirement age are poised to disrupt many long-held plans, promises, assumptions, and expectations about retirement. Two of the biggest issues are whether baby boomers will be able to retire and, if so, when. If baby boomers must continue to work, then their hearing must be sharper than if they were playing golf with friends in Florida.

If we start by considering how well the average baby boomer has been saving for retirement, things look pretty good. The Congressional Budget Office (CBO 2004) reports that the typical baby boomer earns a higher income and has accumulated more wealth than had his or her parents at a similar age. The American Association of Retired Persons (AARP 1994) projects that baby boomers will generally earn more in retirement than current retirees. If we look beyond these averages, however, not everyone does so well. The CBO also reports that a quarter of baby boomers have failed to accumulate significant savings and are likely to depend entirely on government programs for retirement. Another quarter will need to reduce their standard of living. The AARP notes a gradually widening gap between the best-off and worst-off households. In addition, it reports that the lowest-earning 20 percent of baby boomers will receive 80 percent of their income from Social Security.

A number of assumptions go into projecting financial preparedness for retirement. The projections made can vary greatly, depending on the specific assumptions and their accuracy. Demographers made this point by noting that with favorable assumptions, households could be expected to accumulate sufficient wealth for retirement by saving 3–9 percent of their income per year. With different assumptions such as a poor return on investments or longer life expectancy, these savings requirements could increase to as high as 16–29 percent per year (Gist et al. 1999). Taking this variability into account, one study (Gale 1997) concludes that one-third of baby boomers were accumulating sufficient wealth for retirement under any reasonable set of assumptions. Another third will not be financially prepared regardless of the assumptions. The remaining third may or may not have sufficient wealth for retirement. It all depends on how things actually work out.

Government programs that retirees have traditionally relied on such as Social Security and Medicare are likely to be overwhelmed by the number of baby boomers (General Accounting Office 2002). By 2020 one in six Americans will be sixty-five years of age or over. This is 20 million people more than in 2002. At the same time, the ratio of workers paying taxes into these systems compared with retirees drawing benefits will be at an all-time low. Even with Social Security increasing the eligibility age to sixty-seven, the cost of this entitlement is expected to rise. It is difficult to envision a scenario in which these realities will not place limitations on baby boomer benefits.

Although some would look to the stock market as the answer, this is not without its own problems. First, there are obvious risks such as the Enron fiasco or the downturn at the end of the 1990s. The biggest problem arises from the devaluation of assets that will occur when baby boomers sell their stocks to finance their retirement. It is difficult to make a profit from selling when everyone is trying to sell. Looking at all of the information that is available to him today, Harry Dent, the financial guru who predicted the stock market boom of the 1990s, predicts a "bear" market through the majority of baby boomer retirement years. He warns that although he expects stocks to do well from 2005 to 2009, the market will most likely loose value after 2010 (Dent 2004).

Family has traditionally formed at least part of the safety net for many people in their retirement years. Children may help with financial support, a place to live, or disabilities, or they may serve as unpaid caregivers. This support will be less available for many baby boomers because they had fewer children. By 2020 the number of retirees living alone and without family support is expected to be double what it was in 1990 (Siegel 1996). As a result, baby boomers may need to be increasingly self-reliant.

Perhaps it is not surprising that many baby boomers plan to continue working after retirement. The American Association of Retired Persons (AARP 2004) reported that about 80 percent of baby boomers plan to work in some capacity during their retirement years. A growing percentage of post-retirement workers were planning to work out of financial necessity rather than for enjoyment. A survey of Texas baby boomers also found a large number (68 percent) planning to work after retirement (Texas Department on Aging 2000). Currently, just 12 percent of the older population is employed in the Texas workforce.

This may seem like a lot of information about retirement for a book about hearing loss, but it is relevant for baby boomers. How will a boomer cope if he or she develops hearing loss and needs to continue working? Although this dilemma can and does occur to many people before their retirement years, it will become epidemic for elderly baby boomers.

Expectations

Hearing loss may also be problematic for many baby boomers because of their worldview. When Landon Jones titled his 1980 book *Great Expectations*, he was not talking about the text's anticipated sales numbers. He was stressing that baby boomers share something beyond being part of a large group. They share high expectations for their lifestyle. Baby boomers have lived during a very affluent time. They would never have become known as the "me" generation without an underlying affluence to support their self-indulgence. A "me" generation would not have arisen during the Great Depression. Poverty and financial hardship have existed during the baby boom years, but not with the same incidence found in previous generations. The level of financial hardship known by baby boomers has more often involved buying fewer record albums or buying an economy car rather than an expensive import. Baby boomers have had more and expected more. This has been reflected in their spending habits, leisure activities, lifestyle, and sense of entitlement.

Baby boomers have also lived during a time of seemingly unlimited possibilities. They experienced the startling feats of *Sputnik* circling the earth in 1957 and a man walking on the moon in 1969. The transistor was invented in 1948 and was followed a decade later by the integrated circuit. This made possible the computer and information technology revolutions. Medical advances were made in diagnostics, imaging, surgery, microsurgery, cosmetic surgery, transplants, pharmaceuticals, and the like. Regardless of the field, progress seemed to be moving at an ever-increasing pace. Although some people may have felt overwhelmed by these advances, baby boomers were much better prepared to cope and even thrive. They had attained a higher level of education than any previous generation. Nearly 90 percent completed high school, and almost 30 percent completed a college bachelor's degree or higher (U.S. Census Bureau 2000). This education gave baby boomers the tools to better understand and benefit from the progress being made. The progressive atmosphere baby boomers have inhabited has not been one that would prepare them to graciously accept limits.

Hearing loss is an affront to baby boomer expectations. Baby boomers typically see themselves as too young to suffer hearing loss. The existence of hearing loss may instead be seen as a failure of the medical and scientific advances that baby boomers have come to expect. Hearing loss represents unforeseen disability and hardship. It means one may have to do less or settle for less. Although some baby boomers may wish to follow the lead of previous generations and try to ignore hearing loss as a problem, this strategy is impractical and almost guarantees a negative outcome.

Some Final Words about Baby Boomers and Hearing Loss

Although categorizing baby boomers is not really possible, they do share common ground with regard to hearing loss. They are likely to have at least some history of noise exposure. The odds are high that they will live to an age at which hearing loss is most common. Unfortunately that age is quickly approaching. Baby boomers face the prospects of delayed retirement or working through the traditional retirement years, thereby increasing the need for continued good hearing. Aside from the issue of continuing to work in later life, baby boomers may also find that hearing loss shatters some of their leisure and lifestyle expectations. Reduced quality of life becomes a concern.

The good news is that baby boomers who suffer hearing loss have medical, surgical, and technological solutions that were unavailable to previous generations. They are also more likely to have the education to be able to evaluate these options. Even better, the majority of baby boomers still have time before hearing loss is likely to be a problem. That is, it is possible to act now to minimize the risk of developing hearing loss. There is also the chance that new treatments will become available between now and when a hearing loss might occur. What's more, we have the option to support research or other hearing-related programs from which we all might ultimately benefit.

Baby boomers have the chance to take control of—rather than be controlled by—their hearing future. Before choosing a course of action, however, it is best to have a basic understanding of how the ear works and how things can go wrong. This is where we turn next.

3 How the Ear Works

The human ear is a tremendously intricate yet efficient structure. It contains many individual parts interacting in harmony to collect sounds from the outside world and send them to the brain. It works so well that the ear is typically taken for granted. The buzz of a bee, the purr of a cat, and the sound of a symphony orchestra are all perceived as external. The workings of the ear are perceptually transparent.

Although hearing may on the surface appear to be a simple process, it is not. It involves collecting airborne sounds and transmitting them through tissue, bone, and fluids. Sounds must then be converted into electrical impulses that are sent along nerves to be interpreted by the brain. Any little thing that might go wrong along the way can impede or stop the transmission of sound. Considering how much can go wrong, it is not only amazing that the auditory system works but that it works so well.

This chapter examining the human ear is divided into several parts. In the first part, the inner workings of the ear are explained. Discussions of anatomy and function are detailed but not exhaustive. The intent is to provide useful information that will not be overwhelming. In the second part, the system used to classify the different types of hearing loss is presented. Finally, the individual parts of a hearing test are discussed, and the graph of these results—the audiogram—is explained. After reading this chapter you should be able to look at an audiogram and recognize if there is a hearing loss, the severity of the loss, and whether the loss is one that is likely to be medically correctable.

Understanding the Ear

The human ear is shown in figure 3.1. Anatomically the ear is separated into three adjoining parts: the outer ear, the middle ear, and the inner ear.

The Outer Ear

The auricle, ear canal, and eardrum make up the outer ear. The auricle (also called the pinna) is the external part of the ear that can be seen. Contrary to popular opinion, it does more than provide a place to hang eyeglasses or put earrings. The outer ear collects sound and directs it into the ear canal. It is the physiological equivalent of the ear trumpets that were used before the invention of hearing aids. Cartilage provides the structure of the auricle, and all of the curves and ridges help to give it strength while allowing some flexibility. The shape may seem odd, but it is very functional.

The ear canal extends from the auricle to the eardrum. In most people it is about one inch in length. The course of the ear canal is slightly curved and is a bit lower at the outer entrance than at the eardrum. This sloping helps prevent water or debris from accumulating in the canal. The outer portion of the canal is supported by cartilage and then bone farther in the ear. The outer portion of the ear canal is also home to some hair cells and ceruminous cells that produce earwax. Both may serve a protective function. Hair in the canal can block insects from entering. Cerumen helps to keep the skin of the canal slightly acidic, which may help to prevent bacterial or fungal growth.

The eardrum serves as the innermost end to the ear canal. It is known medically as the tympanic membrane. This membrane is the barrier between the outer and middle ear. Situated on the border, the eardrum might be considered as part of either the outer or middle ear. Convention holds, however, that it be considered part of the middle ear. The rationale behind this convention is that sound traverses the auricle and ear canal through the vibration of air molecules. At the eardrum and through the middle ear it is body structures—the eardrum and ear bones—that are vibrating to transmit sound. It makes more sense to classify the eardrum with the middle ear because

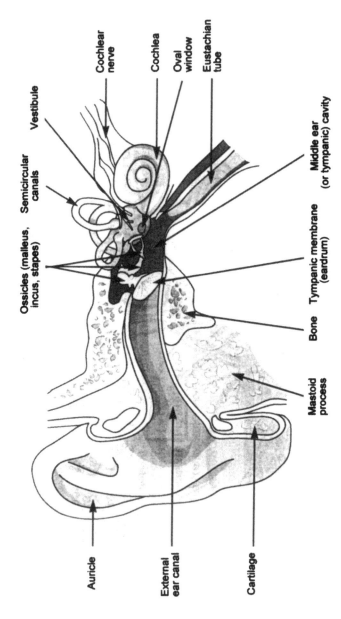

Figure 3.1. *The human ear. Courtesy of the Society of Otorhinolaryngology and Head-Neck Nurses (www.sohnnurse.com)*

Cochlear nerve

Cochlea

Oval window

Eustachian tube

Vestibule

Semicircular canals

Ossicles (malleus, incus, stapes)

Middle ear (or tympanic) cavity

Tympanic membrane (eardrum)

Bone

Mastoid process

Auricle

External ear canal

Cartilage

the mode of sound transmission has changed. The eardrum is considered further during the discussion of the middle ear.

The auricle and ear canal serve as more than a conduit for sound because they also modify it. Just as low-pitched sounds resonate well in a tuba or middle-pitched sounds are produced by a trumpet, high-pitched sounds are emphasized in the small space of the ear canal. The amplifying effect of the ear canal was calculated as early as the late 1930s (Flemming 1939). In 1960 physicist Georg von Bekesy was able to clinically measure this amplifying effect along with the subtle variations produced by the interaction of the eardrum. The total high-frequency boost is enough that, without it, our language might need to contain fewer speech sounds. Quiet high-pitched sounds such as *f* or *th* would be inaudible.

The Middle Ear

The primary structures of the middle ear are shown in figure 3.2. They include the eardrum and ear bones (ossicles). The eardrum forms the outside boundary of the middle ear. Attached to the eardrum is the outermost of the ossicles—the malleus. The inner end of the malleus connects to the incus bone, which in turn connects to

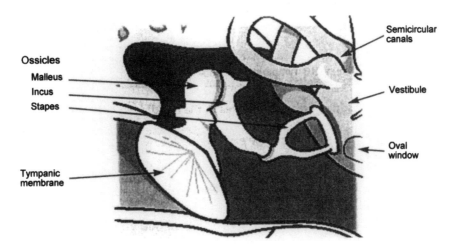

Figure 3.2. The middle ear. Courtesy of the Society of Otorhinolaryngology and Head-Neck Nurses (www.sohnnurse.com)

the stapes bone. The ossicles are also known respectively as the hammer, anvil, and stirrup. The innermost end of the stapes (the footplate) rests in the oval window, which serves as the opening to the inner ear. Several ligaments suspend the ossicles within the middle ear cavity. This cavity has a volume of one or two cubic centimeters and is filled with air. The ligaments allow the ossicles to move freely, transferring sound through the middle ear.

The eardrum is about a quarter inch across. It is shaped like the cone of a loud speaker extending slightly into the middle ear at the center. A healthy eardrum is translucent and has a pearly gray color. Although the eardrum is very thin and lightweight, it is made up of three different layers of tissue. It is the fibrous center layer that gives the eardrum its strength and resilience. Aside from serving as a protective barrier to the middle ear, the eardrum absorbs incoming sound and transfers it to the malleus.

The structures of the middle ear serve as more than an odd-looking sound conduit. Their primary role is to prevent sound energy from being lost as it is transferred from the air in the outside world and outer ear to the fluids in the inner ear. Although sound travels well through both air and water, it does not travel well between air and water. If you were to swim underwater in a pool, you likely would have difficulty hearing and understanding the speech of a person who is above the surface. Similarly, if you were in a small boat on the surface of the ocean, it is unlikely you would hear the sounds of whales that are under the surface. Too much of the sound is reflected back or lost between mediums. Without the middle ear, we would hear no better than if we were underwater.

The middle ear acts in two ways to efficiently transition sound from the air to the fluids in the inner ear. The first is by collecting sound at the eardrum and then focusing all of this energy onto the much smaller space of the stapes footplate. This increases the available sound power per area. Power is also preserved by the eardrum and ossicles working together in a lever action. Just as a child sitting at the end of a seesaw can lift an adult sitting closer to the fulcrum, the fortuitous movement of the ossicles increases the sound pressure at the stapes. The net effect is a good transfer of sound from the outside air to the fluids of the inner ear.

One final structure of note in the middle ear is the Eustachian tube. This small passageway leads from the middle ear to an area behind the nasal cavity and above the back portion of the roof of the mouth. It equalizes the pressure between the middle ear and outside world. We have all noticed the pressure imbalance that can occur as we fly in an airplane, drive in the mountains, or dive underwater. It is air passing through the Eustachian tube that keeps the middle ear pressure consistent with our surroundings.

The Inner Ear

The inner ear serves two functions: hearing and balance. The part responsible for hearing is called the cochlea. The part responsible for balance includes the semicircular canals and vestibule. Together the balance portions of the inner ear are known as the vestibular system. The cochlea and vestibular system are shown in figure 3.1.

The cochlea is a small snail-shaped structure that spirals about two and a half turns from the base to the apex. Thousands of nerve cells extend the inside length of the cochlea and are aligned into four rows: one row of inner nerve cells and three rows of outer nerve cells. Small hairs (cilia) extend from the top of the sensory cells, which is why these sensory nerves are also known as hair cells.

Unlike the middle ear, the cochlea is a fluid-filled structure. Sound is transferred to the fluids of the inner ear through the oval window at the base of the cochlea. As the fluid moves, a shearing force is created across the hair at the top of each nerve cell. The nerve cell then fires an electrical signal (sound) along the cochlear nerve to the brain. The mechanical properties of the cochlea cause the nerve cells to be tuned to specific frequencies. Nerve cells close to the base where sound enters the ear fire in response to high-pitched sounds. Moving farther into the cochlea, nerve cells fire in response to lower and lower frequencies. Contemporary experts believe that the majority of sound reaching the brain comes from the inner hair cells and that the outer hair cells act more to enhance the mechanical motion or fluid dynamics within the ear. What is certain is that both inner and outer hair cells are necessary for good hearing.

Our sense of balance is controlled primarily by the vestibular system. We use our vision and feedback from the muscles in our legs to help with balance and orientation, but it is the vestibular system that is in control. Like the cochlea, the structures of the vestibular system are fluid filled. Changes in position are detected by fluid movement, and positional orientation is determined by the pull of gravity. The semicircular canals detect rotational movement such as leaning forward or turning right or left. The vestibule contains the utricle and saccule, which detect linear acceleration. Although the vestibular system is not responsible for hearing, I mention it here because some medical conditions that affect balance also affect hearing.

Understanding the Types of Hearing Loss

There are many causes of hearing loss. Earwax, infection, disease, heredity, trauma, and noise exposure are but a few of the possible causes. Hearing losses also come in varying severities. One person may have a slight hearing loss that is little more than a nuisance while another may have a substantial loss that is very handicapping. The pattern of hearing loss (low pitched versus high pitched) can vary from person to person, as can the ear's ability to process sound. Some people suffering hearing loss will recover on their own, while others require medical or surgical intervention. A large percentage of hearing losses are permanent. The majority of these can be helped by hearing aids, but a few cannot. All of the potential variables associated with hearing problems make the handicap hard to classify.

The most obvious choice would be to classify hearing loss on the basis of cause. This might work with hearing losses resulting from age, heredity, or trauma but presents a serious problem when the underlying cause is unknown, which is quite frequent. This form of classification does not convey the severity of a loss or whether it is medically correctable. A traumatic hearing loss resulting from falling off a roof could be slight or severe. It might be permanent or surgically treatable. Furthermore, the hearing loss suffered by one person falling off a roof can be entirely different from that of another person who experiences a similar fall. Cause by itself does not serve as a particularly helpful classification for hearing loss. Trying to categorize hearing loss primarily in terms of severity, pattern, permanence, or hearing aid candidacy presents similar problems.

The generally accepted scheme for classification involves dividing hearing loss into several types, based on the site of the problem. Founding the method of categorization on location has several advantages. Unlike cause, the site of a hearing loss can always be determined. Also this method makes the classification very concrete. There is no ambiguity. The third advantage is that it provides an indication of whether the loss is correctable or permanent since a problem with certain parts of the ear is much more treatable than a problem in other parts of the ear. Cause, severity, and pattern of hearing loss are still important classifications, but location of the loss is the first consideration.

The three primary types of hearing loss are conductive, sensorineural, and mixed. There is a forth type of hearing loss termed central, but this classification is often treated separately since the site of the hearing problem is not in the ear. Each of these hearing loss types is described in the sections that follow.

Conductive

A hearing loss is considered conductive when there is an impediment to the conduction of sound through the outer or middle ear: either the sound is blocked or the structures of the ear fail to convey the noise. One of the most common causes of a conductive hearing loss is earwax blocking the ear canal. The wax acts as a barrier to sound. Infection in the outer or middle ear can also block sound. A torn eardrum or damaged ossicles can produce a similar hearing loss by failing to convey sound. All of these are examples of a conductive hearing loss.

Conductive hearing losses are the most treatable type. They are usually caused by a diagnosable physical problem that can be medically or surgically corrected: earwax can be removed, infection can be cured, and a damaged eardrum or ear bone can be repaired. In cases in which the damage causing a conductive loss is very severe and cannot be completely corrected, it may still be possible to improve the hearing. Only rarely can a conductive hearing loss not be improved. This diagnosis offers the hope that something can be done.

Sensorineural

A sensorineural hearing loss is what is commonly referred to as a nerve hearing loss. This loss exists when there is damage to the hair cells within the cochlea; they no longer sense the fluid movements within the inner ear, and thus no signal is sent to the brain. A minimal amount of damage involving few nerve cells may result in a mild hearing loss. Greater damage involving more cells produces a greater hearing decrement. This damage can also cause sounds to be distorted. For music listening this can result in a loss of tonality. For speech it can cause problems with understanding. Two of the most common examples of a sensorineural hearing loss are those caused by noise exposure and aging. Both result in damage to the sensory cells of the ear. Unfortunately, unlike conductive hearing losses, sensorineural hearing losses are not usually medically or surgically correctable.

Mixed

When there is both a conductive and sensorineural hearing loss in the same ear, it is classified as a mixed hearing loss. The prognosis for this kind of loss is, as one would expect, mixed. The portion of hearing loss that is conductive is likely to be medically treatable, whereas the portion that is sensorineural is not. This means that the hearing level for a person with a mixed hearing loss can usually be improved but not completely corrected. An example of a mixed hearing loss would be wax blocking an ear that has an underlying nerve hearing loss. The portion of hearing loss resulting from earwax can be corrected by removing the wax. The underlying nerve loss will remain.

Central

Hearing difficulties are termed central when the underlying problem is in the brain or in the nerve pathways leading to the brain. Unlike conductive, sensorineural, and mixed hearing losses, a central hearing loss does not usually result in a loss of hearing sensitivity. The problem here is one of understanding. The ears send a clear message to the brain, but the brain has difficulty making sense of it. Some people are born with a central hearing problem. In school it can cause learning difficulties, and in later life it often appears as a lack of attention. Brain damage from a stroke, car accident, or trauma is another cause of central hearing loss that is acquired in adulthood.

Upon learning the description of central hearing loss, many people with hearing problems incorrectly conclude that this describes them. In the vast majority of cases a person fails to understand not because the brain cannot process sound but rather because the ears do not send it. People with relatively mild hearing losses can easily be fooled into believing their problem is neurological not auditory since they hear others talking but don't understand them. These people don't realize that even a slight hearing loss is enough to prevent them from hearing some of the softer consonant sounds. They have difficulty understanding because there are letters missing. People also mistake the distortion from a sensorineural hearing loss occurring within the ear as originating within the brain.

Central auditory problems do occur and can be handicapping. They are, however, less common than conductive, sensorineural, and mixed losses. When someone complains to a hearing professional about difficulty understanding, the professional almost always starts by first looking for one of these more likely causes.

Understanding a Hearing Test

The standard hearing test is a powerful but underappreciated tool both descriptively and diagnostically. There is more to it than listening for a series of beeps. To understand a hearing test, it helps to know all of the things that can be learned from the results. Second, it helps to know the different parts of the test. A hearing test involves not just one task but instead consists of several tests grouped together. Finally, it is important to know how to interpret the audiogram, a graph of the hearing test results.

What Can Be Learned from a Hearing Test

The most obvious thing that can be learned from a hearing test is a person's hearing sensitivity, that is, the softest volume at which someone can hear a range of sounds. This measure can be used to rule out, confirm, or quantify a hearing loss. It can also be compared to previous tests to check for any changes in hearing. In most people's minds this is where the value of a hearing test ends. What is not understood is that a hearing test additionally measures the clarity of hearing. Knowing how soft a sound a person can hear provides an incomplete picture without also knowing how well that person can understand what is heard.

The diagnostic value of a hearing test often goes unrecognized as well. Certain patterns of hearing loss serve as an indicator or signature of specific ear diseases and pathologies. There are hearing-impaired ears that look absolutely normal to an ear doctor and are diagnosed on the basis of the hearing test results. Additionally, the hearing test classifies a hearing loss as conductive, sensorineural, or mixed. Because the potential for hearing improvement is directly related to the amount of hearing loss that is found to be conductive, hearing test results weigh heavily in most decisions regarding ear surgery.

Parts of a Hearing Test

The typical hearing test is made up of four subtests. Collectively they are known as the audiometric test battery. The four parts are air conduction, bone conduction, speech reception threshold, and word discrimination. Each is discussed in turn.

Air conduction testing. Air conduction testing is the part most people associate with having a hearing test. The person being tested listens for tones (beeps) through headphones. His or her task is to respond (push a button, raise a hand, and so forth) whenever a tone is heard. The tester records the quietest level to which the person consistently responds at a variety of pitches. These are the listener's hearing thresholds. Because the test equipment is calibrated to a national standard, the test results are comparable between hearing centers and over time. Results from a hearing test performed in Dallas, Texas, fifteen years ago can be compared with results from a test performed today in Kalamazoo, Michigan.

Bone conduction testing. Bone conduction testing is done in a similar way to air conduction testing, but the tones are not presented using a standard headphone. Instead, a small bone vibrator is worn behind the ear on the mastoid bone. This device gently vibrates the skull and sends the tones through the skull directly to the inner ear.

Although this may sound bizarre, it is essentially the way you hear your own voice. The vibration of your vocal chords transfers to your skull and goes to the inner ear. This direct sound route explains why your voice sounds different to you live than it does on tape. When speaking aloud you hear yourself through this direct route. On tape, the sound you hear is shaped by the resonance of the outer ear.

Bone conduction testing is valuable because it provides a direct measure of the hearing sensitivity of the inner ear. It completely bypasses the outer and middle ear and is different from air conduction and speech measures that test the entire auditory system. If a person hears better through bone conduction than by air conduction, sound is being lost in the outer or middle ear. This is a conductive hearing loss. Subtracting the bone conduction threshold from the air conduction threshold (the air–bone gap) shows exactly how much sound is lost. If the air and bone conduction scores are the same, then no sound is being lost on the way to the inner ear. Consequently, any hearing loss that is found must instead be in the inner ear and therefore sensorineural.

Speech reception threshold testing. The speech reception threshold (SRT) is the lowest level that a person is able to hear and at which he or she can identify two-syllable words. The required task for the person being tested is simply to repeat as many of the two-syllable words as possible until the words become inaudible to the test taker. The volume at which the words are presented is monitored through calibrated equipment so that the results are accurate and comparable to pure tone thresholds.

Word discrimination score testing. The task for the person being tested in word discrimination score (WDS) testing is also to repeat as many words as possible. The difference from SRT testing is that the words are presented well above a person's hearing threshold. Another difference is that in WDS testing, the percentage of correct answers is recorded. The first is a measure of sensitivity, and the second is a measure of clarity. The goal in WDS testing is to determine the best a person can understand under ideal conditions.

The words used are specially selected to provide a representative mix of all of the speech sounds in a particular language. Different lists exist for different languages. Because the word lists are standard-ized and the presentation level recorded, discrimination scores are comparable over time and between hearing centers.

Reading an Audiogram

Figure 3.3 shows a typical audiogram. Sound frequency (pitch) is shown on the x-axis, and sound intensity (loudness) is shown on the y-axis. Symbols toward the top of the graph indicate the ability to hear quiet sounds. Symbols farther down the graph indicate sounds not being heard until they are louder. (The symbols are explained further in box 3.1.) Low-pitched sounds are represented on the left side of the graph and higher pitches on the right. If after looking at the placement of the symbols in figure 3.3 you conclude that this per-son must have pretty good hearing, you would be right. This is the audiogram of a person with normal hearing thresholds.

The frequency distribution at the bottom of the graph usually seems odd to anyone not accustomed to looking at an audiogram.

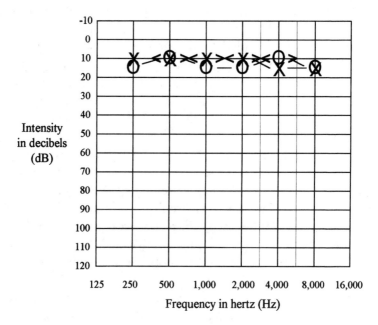

Figure 3.3. Audiogram showing normal hearing.

Most people understand that frequency is measured in hertz (Hz), which is the number of cycles or sound waves per second. The problem is that the numbers do not progress in a linear fashion. Instead, the frequency doubles with each line on the graph. Frequencies are plotted this way because perceptually, the human ear follows this pattern. Every doubling or halving in frequency is perceived as a one-octave change. Changing from 250 Hz to 500 Hz is one octave, just as changing from 4,000 Hz to 8,000 Hz is one octave. Thinking in terms of octaves explains the numbers.

The other aspect that may seem odd about the included frequencies is that they do not cover the full human hearing range of 20–20,000 Hz. The frequencies on an audiogram are biased to represent those that are most needed to hear and understand speech. These sounds generally range between 500 Hz and 4,000 Hz. Adding one octave on either end gives us the 250–8,000 Hz range that is included on most audiograms. Although it is possible to test beyond these limits, it is not usually necessary.

The y-axis of the audiogram appears more orderly than the x-axis. The numbers proceed in a linear manner, leading one to conclude that a threshold marked at 50 might be 20 percent worse than a threshold marked at 30. However, it's not so simple. The units of measurement on the y-axis are called decibels (dB) and act logarithmically, meaning that they grow exponentially rather than linearly. Zero on this scale is not the absence of sound. Rather, it is the softest level the average person can hear under ideal conditions. Sound levels grow at an increasingly faster rate from here. At 20 dB the sound pressure is ten times greater than at 0 dB. At 40 dB it is one hundred times greater than at 0 dB. By 120 dB the sound pressure is one million times greater. Processing this enormous pressure differential may seem impossible, but it is what allows the human ear to detect as little energy as the sound produced by the wings of a gnat or as much as is produced by the sound of a jet airliner taking off. Fortunately, this rapid increase in sound pressure is not perceived so abruptly. The ear interprets the exponential progression in volume as being linear. A sound increase of one decibel is perceived as the same change in volume, whether it is from 20 dB to 21 dB or from 70 dB to 71 dB. The decibel scale takes into account our perception of loudness while providing a simple way to quantify the intensity of sound.

The most common symbols used on an audiogram are shown in box 3.1. All of the symbols representing the right ear are usually drawn in red, and symbols representing the left ear are drawn in blue. At times during a hearing test there is the risk that sound intended to be heard in one ear might instead be heard in the other. To prevent this, an examiner might add a whooshing or shower-like sound to the ear not being tested. Adding this sound to the nontest ear does not affect the threshold of the ear being tested or affects it only negligibly. As shown in box 3.1, different threshold symbols are used to indicate when masking sound is being added to the opposite ear.

The severity of hearing loss can be expressed in terms of decibels (i.e., a 30- or 40-dB loss). Most nonprofessionals, however, tend to treat these numbers as percentages. Although technically wrong, it is descriptive. Larger numbers represent a greater amount of hearing loss, and by the time 100 dB (100 percent) is reached, a hearing loss is severe enough to appear total even when some usable hearing may remain. Somewhere between the technically correct and mathematically inaccurate is the simplification that is most commonly used. The decibel remains the basis of this classification strategy, but the amount of loss is expressed in more understandable terms, such as *mild* or *severe*. The complete description of this scheme is shown in box 3.2.

Box 3.1. Audiometric symbols

	Right ear	*Left ear*
Hearing threshold	◯	X
Masked hearing threshold*	△	☐
Bone conduction threshold	<	>
Masked bone conduction threshold*	[	]

*Masking noise is introduced into the opposite ear to prevent it from helping the ear being tested

---

Box 3.2. Hearing loss severity scale

Normal hearing	0–20 dB
Mild loss	20–40 dB
Moderate loss	40–60 dB
Moderately severe loss	60–80 dB
Severe loss	80–100 dB
Profound loss	100–120 dB

Word discrimination and speech reception threshold results are not usually written onto the audiogram graph. They are instead written below or to the side of the audiogram. The word discrimination score heading might be abbreviated as DISC or WDS. It is alternately referred to as a word recognition score, or WRS.

Putting It All Together

One example of a normal audiogram is insufficient to bring together the many issues discussed in this chapter because it neither shows how a sensorineural loss will appear on an audiogram nor illustrates how to recognize a loss that might be medically correctable. Therefore we consider a few more examples, including audiograms of sensorineural, conductive, and mixed hearing loss. The issue of word understanding is also discussed in relation to these hearing losses.

Example of a conductive hearing loss. The audiogram in figure 3.4 shows normal hearing in the left ear and a conductive hearing loss in the right ear. The left ear is normal because all of the air and bone conduction thresholds for that ear are above 20 dB. Note that there is no gap between the air and bone conduction thresholds in this ear. This indicates that no sound is being lost as it passes through the outer or middle ear.

The right ear is a different story. Although the bone conduction thresholds are essentially normal, air conduction thresholds show about a 40-dB hearing loss. The good bone conduction scores indicate that the hearing nerves in the inner ear work well. The problem is the 15- to 30-dB gap between the air and bone conduction thresholds.

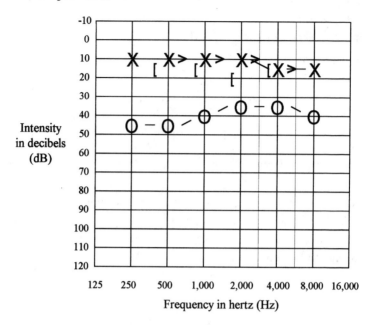

Figure 3.4. Audiogram showing a conductive hearing loss.

This is the amount of sound being lost in the outer or middle ear. This is also the amount of loss that may be medically correctable. In other words, the hearing in this ear has the potential to be brought back to normal.

Example of a sensorineural hearing loss. The audiogram shown in figure 3.5 is entirely different from the previous one. This would typically be described as a bilateral-sloping mild-to-severe sensorineural hearing loss. In this case there is no air–bone gap. The outer and middle ear work fine. The depressed bone conduction thresholds show that the problem is in the inner ear. This is not a hearing loss that is likely to be corrected medically.

Example of a mixed hearing loss. A severe mixed hearing loss is shown in figure 3.6. This graph shows neither the conductive or sensory portions of either ear to be working well. The bone conduction thresholds for the right ear are at about 35 dB and for the left ear at 55 dB. Aside from indicating nerve loss, the audiogram shows an additional conductive component of 20 dB in the left ear and 35–45 dB

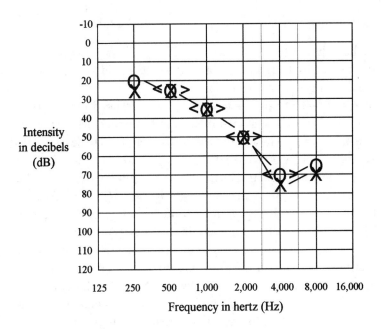

Figure 3.5. Audiogram showing a sensorineural hearing loss.

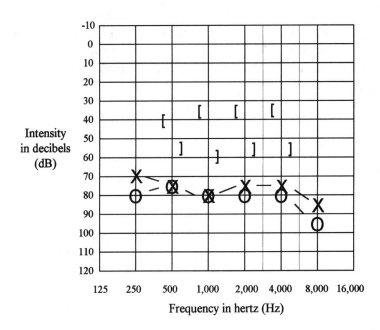

Figure 3.6. Audiogram showing a mixed hearing loss.

in the right ear. In the best scenario, it might be possible to improve the hearing in the right ear from a severe to a mild loss and to bring the left ear up to a moderate loss.

A word about word understanding. As explained previously, audiometric thresholds alone provide an incomplete description of a person's hearing. The ability to understand also has to be considered. Although poor word understanding scores would be atypical for a person with a conductive hearing loss, it is still important that they be measured to ensure that nothing is missed. Word understanding becomes a greater issue with mixed and sensorineural hearing losses. The nerve damage that is present in these cases can greatly impact a person's ability to understand under even the best conditions. Furthermore, the amount of word understanding difficulty cannot be accurately predicted for an individual on the basis of his or her hearing thresholds. Word understanding has to be measured in each case.

Word comprehension also has relevance in regard to treatment options. Surgically correcting the conductive portion of the mixed loss shown in figure 3.6 may be of little value if the underlying cause for the sensorineural portion was one that left the inner ear or auditory nerve that leads to the brain unable to process speech. Similarly, hearing aids may be of great or little value in compensating for the sensorineural hearing loss shown in figure 3.5. In these instances and many others, knowing a person's word understanding ability is key.

Now that we understand anatomy and function in addition to hearing thresholds and word understanding, its time to explain the causes and treatments for hearing loss.

4 Causes and Treatments for Hearing Loss

There are many causes of hearing loss. A review of them all would be extremely complicated and require many more pages than are in this book. Even the best hearing professionals often require reference texts, medical journals, or a good research library to keep abreast of some of the more obscure diseases and syndromes. Our task of understanding the causes of hearing loss need not be so daunting, however, because only a handful of causes are responsible for the vast majority of hearing losses. These are the focus of this chapter. They are organized on the basis of whether the loss is preventable, treatable, or in some way surmountable.

Preventable Hearing Loss

True to the old adage, prevention is the best cure. This is good news for most baby boomers, many of whom are still young enough to stave off a preventable hearing problem through simple lifestyle changes. Even a person who has already sustained a hearing loss may be able to halt it at an early stage. Previous generations were often unaware of many risks to their hearing and sometimes dismissed the ones that were known. They also tended to ignore a developing hearing problem until it presented a significant impediment. Baby boomers have the opportunity to do better. They have more information on which to act and time remaining to do so.

Some causes of preventable hearing loss are easy to steer clear of. Others may be difficult or impossible to avoid. Even in these cases, however, it is usually possible to minimize their effects.

Noise Exposure

Noise exposure is responsible for the majority of preventable hearing losses. Loud sounds can so overdrive the structures in the ear that trauma results. In extreme cases such as an explosion, the eardrum can be torn or the ossicles broken or displaced. More commonly it is the delicate nerve cells in the inner ear that are damaged. Once the nerves are damaged, the resulting hearing loss is permanent. Because the nerve endings for high frequencies are first in line as sound enters the inner ear, the majority of sound trauma occurs here, resulting in high-frequency hearing loss. With long-term noise exposure, however, all of the frequencies can be affected.

Initially, exposure to loud sound may only cause a temporary hearing loss known as a temporary threshold shift (TTS). This short-term phenomenon typically produces a hearing impairment that is mild, but the loss can be more severe. If you ever noticed your hearing reduced for a short time after cutting the grass or attending a rock concert, you have likely experienced TTS. Sounds will appear softer than normal for a time, or TTS may instead make your ears feel like they are full or plugged. This should serve as a warning because with repeated exposure sounds that are loud enough to cause TTS can eventually result in a permanent thresholds shift (PTS).

The risk of hearing damage from loud sound has been recognized in industry for many years. In 1969 the Walsh-Healey Act placed limits on acceptable noise exposure in the workplace. The allowable level was based on the intensity of sound and the length of exposure. Continuous exposure to 90 dB was allowed for no more than eight hours per day. For every 5-dB increase in loudness beyond this level, a 50 percent reduction in the total time exposed was required (i.e., four hours at 95 dB, two hours at 100 dB, and so forth). The industrial noise standards today require workers to wear hearing protection (earplugs or earmuffs) if they are exposed to unsafe noise levels. Sound intensity is tested in the workplace in order to know which workers may be at risk. At-risk workers are also required to have yearly hearing tests to ensure that the noise isn't damaging their hearing (U.S. Department of Labor 1989). These rules have protected the hearing of countless workers, but many small businesses have never had their noise levels checked for safety, and many workers fail to wear hearing protection despite warnings.

Industrial noise and loud music are not the only causes of noise-induced hearing loss. Other potential sources are listed in box 4.1. Few would be surprised to hear that professional soldiers have been found to suffer severe hearing deterioration from gunfire (Ylikoski 1994). What is less well appreciated is that similar results have been documented in recreational shooters (Nondahl et al. 2000). Picturesque farmlands might seem an unlikely place to develop a noise-induced hearing loss, but the equipment used there poses a significant hearing risk to farmers (Plakke and Dare 1992). Audiologists found the risk from leisure-time noise exposure to be similar to that of exposure to noise in industrial settings (Dalton et al. 2001). Those who engage in leisure activities involving noise levels greater than 90 dB were found to have an increased incidence of hearing loss. The amount of loss increased with years of exposure. Leisure-time woodworkers, for example, were 30 percent more likely to have hearing loss than were non-woodworkers.

Without the benefit of posted sound levels it can be difficult to recognize the situations that pose a hearing risk. One way to solve this problem would be to buy a sound-level meter. These can sometimes be purchased inexpensively from a local electronics store. The use of certain environmental and situational indicators is another approach employed for years in industry. Difficulty communicating because of the noise, or experiencing head noise or TTS after

---

Box 4.1. A few potentially damaging sources of noise

Air compressors	Fireworks	Nightclubs
Auto racing	Gasoline string trimmers	Power tools
Chain saws	Hairdryers	Rock concerts
Carpet cleaners	Home stereos	Shooting
Car radios	Lawnmowers	Snow blowers
Construction work	Leaf blowers	Tractor pulls
Factory work	Motorcycles	Vacuum cleaners
Farm equipment	Musical instruments	Watercraft

noise exposure are two of these indicators (American Academy of Otolaryngology–Head and Neck Surgery Foundation 1982). If these clues are present, you may be at risk of hearing damage.

The surest way to prevent a noise-induced hearing loss is to avoid loud noise. When this is not possible, sound-blocking earplugs or earmuffs can provide protection. Earplugs and muffs can be purchased inexpensively from a hardware, home improvement, or gun store. If your noise exposure is work related, your employer should provide this protection. Earplugs and earmuffs are rated in decibels by how much sound is attenuated. The bigger the number, the better. A rating of 25–30 dB is sufficient for most situations. Periodic hearing tests can ensure that these measures are adequate to protect your hearing. A decline in hearing would indicate the need for better protection. Please note that putting cotton in the ears offers little or no hearing protection.

Smoking

The increased risk of hearing loss is yet another reason not to smoke. Although the risk of sensorineural hearing damage from smoking is not nearly as high as it is from noise exposure, it is still significant (Palmer et al. 2004). Smokers are about twice as likely to develop hearing loss as nonsmokers (Cruickshanks, Klein, et al. 1998; Itoh et al. 2001; Sharabi et al. 2002). Given all of the known toxins in cigarette smoke, it should not be surprising that some of them might gradually poison the sensory cells in the inner ear. Perhaps most disconcerting is the finding that nonsmokers who live with a smoker are also twice as likely to develop hearing loss (Cruickshanks, Klein, et al. 1998). On the basis of these findings, it is reasonable to conclude that never smoking or quitting smoking may reduce not only your own chance of developing hearing loss but also the chances of those around you.

High Blood Pressure

An increase in the incidence and severity of sensorineural hearing loss has been linked to high blood pressure (Talbott et al. 1990; Gates et al. 1993; Brant et al. 1996; Pirodda et al. 1999). Medical researchers found that high blood pressure affected not only hearing thresholds but also word understanding (Talbott et al. 1990). The relation was strong enough that they proposed using hearing loss as a possible marker for high blood pressure. The cause of hearing loss from high blood pressure is most likely damage to the microvascular blood supply of the ear. Researchers have suggested that preventing or controlling high blood pressure might be a way to avoid many hearing losses that are now attributed to age (Brant et al. 1996).

Diabetes

Hearing loss has also been associated with diabetes. A large-scale study comparing the hearing of more than 12,000 diabetic patients with that of over 50,000 nondiabetic patients found the incidence of sensorineural hearing loss to be greater among the diabetic patients (Kakarlapudi et al. 2003). Furthermore, they found that poor control of the disease was associated with worse hearing. The loss was attributed both to the same microvascular damage that occurs with high blood pressure and to atrophy of the hair cells and cochlear nerve. Ultimately, a diet or lifestyle that reduces your risk of developing diabetes may ultimately reduce your risk of developing hearing loss.

Toxic Medications

Most if not all medications have side effects. Toxicity to the inner ear (ototoxicity), thus causing sensorineural hearing loss, is one potential side effect of some medications. The list of medications that are recognized as potentially damaging to the ear is long and growing. Most people are not surprised to hear that some chemotherapy drugs or powerful antibiotics can damage hearing. There are many other pharmaceuticals, however, that can also pose a hearing risk. Even a medication such as Motrin, which is generally perceived as benign, has a possible association with hearing loss in a very small percentage of people (*Physicians' Desk Reference* 2004). The information needed to protect yourself from ototoxic medications is readily available from a local pharmacist or the *Physicians' Desk Reference*. This resource is updated yearly and provides detailed information on medications. It should be available for review at a local library.

In most instances of medications reported as a possible cause of hearing loss, the risk to the patient's hearing is low, but the patient needs to be aware of any hearing change while on one of these medications and to contact a doctor immediately if he or she notices a difference. Discontinuation, a change in dosage, or an alternate medication may be in order. Periodic hearing tests can also be performed to monitor any changes in hearing. If need be, it is often possible to replace a potentially ototoxic medication with a different, non-ototoxic one.

Toxic Substances

Medicines are not the only ototoxic concern. Various industrial solvents have long been known to cause hearing loss (Rybak 1992). A few of the known offenders include trichloroethylene, xylene, styrene, and carbon monoxide. Trichloroethylene has been used as a degreaser, dry cleaning solvent, and an additive to paint, pesticides, and other products. Xylene has been added to paint, varnishes, and paint thinners. Styrene is used in the manufacture of plastic. Carbon monoxide is everywhere. Rybak additionally explains that the heavy metals arsenic, mercury, lead, tin, and manganese can also be ototoxic in the human body. The problem of ototoxicity is compounded when combined with exposure to loud noise (Morata and Little 2002; Sliwinska-Kowalska et al. 2003).

Although the last paragraph frames ototoxicity in an industrial context, it is not just a work-related problem. Paints and varnishes are used in the home. Assorted cleaners are used in the kitchen and bathroom. Pesticides are used on the lawn. Until recently, arsenic was used in pressure-treated lumber. The average person likely uses a wider array of solvents and chemical solutions in the home than at work. Some of these have the potential to be ototoxic. Their combined effect on hearing is unknown.

You can protect yourself by being aware of the problem. If you work in a job that requires the use of potentially toxic solvents, use adequate ventilation, a ventilated hood, a mask, or breathing apparatus to protect yourself. When the label on a paint can at home says to use with adequate ventilation, use it with more than adequate ventilation. Wear gloves when working with chemicals or solvents that may be absorbed through the skin. Read the labels on all of the cleaners and solvents you use. Few labels will specifically mention hearing.

Watch out though if they mention words such as *neural damage, toxicity, poison, seizure, hazard,* or *death.* Hearing loss may be an omitted footnote to these. Avoid or limit exposure to chemicals you do not know to be safe. As with noise exposure or ototoxic medicines, periodic audiograms can be performed to monitor hearing.

Any factor that poses a threat to your ears must also be viewed as a potential threat to other somatic systems. By protecting your ears, you may be protecting other structures and functions as well.

Treatable Hearing Loss

If you already have a hearing loss, the focus of your interest has likely shifted from prevention to treatment options. Although not all hearing losses can be treated medically or surgically, some can. Your task at this point is to discover if your loss is one of these and to consult with a doctor or audiologist.

Professional involvement is also a good idea even if you do not feel the hearing loss to be bad enough to require care. By seeking immediate care, you may learn of treatment options or other measures that might prevent your hearing from becoming worse. Professional consultation can also serve to rule out hearing loss as a symptom of a larger problem. Box 4.2 lists a number of ear-related symptoms that should serve as a red flag, indicating the need for a medical evaluation.

Box 4.2. Symptoms indicating the need for a medical evaluation

1. Ear pain
2. Drainage from the ear
3. An odor coming from the ear
4. Dizziness
5. Fluctuating hearing
6. Hearing that is worse in one ear than the other
7. Tinnitus (ringing) that is worse in one ear than the other
8. A rapidly progressive hearing loss
9. A sudden hearing loss

Audiologists and otologists are the professionals expressly trained to deal with ear and hearing problems. Audiologists are specialists in hearing science and have earned a master's or doctoral degree from an accredited university. They evaluate patient histories, perform and interpret ear-related tests, dispense hearing aids, provide rehabilitative services, and refer patients to a physician when medical or surgical treatment is needed.

An otologist is a specialized physician who works only with ear problems. An ear, nose, and throat (ENT) physician, known as an otorhinolaryngologist, works with the nose and throat in addition to the ear. If medication or surgery can preserve or improve your hearing, these are the professionals to see. The sections that follow discuss some of the more common ear and hearing problems that are treatable by otologists and ENT physicians.

Earwax

In terms of hearing, earwax only becomes a problem if it completely blocks the ear canal or presses up against the eardrum, thus inhibiting its movement. If either of these conditions occurs, a significant conductive hearing impediment can result. A nonprescription earwax removal system available at drugstores is frequently effective in eliminating this wax. If this is not effective, a general practitioner, audiologist, or other health professional may be able to remove the wax during an office visit. The person best equipped to remove earwax, however, is usually an otologist or ENT physician. They have the tools to remove the buildup from small, narrow, or oddly shaped ear canals.

Interestingly, an earwax problem is often self-inflicted by an overzealous person armed with a cotton swab who pushes the wax farther into the ear and up against the eardrum. An improperly used ear wash can also cause problems. If the wash only softens but does not remove the accumulation, the wax may form a hardened ball that blocks the ear canal once it dries. Keep in mind that a little earwax is normal and does not need to be removed from the canals. If a person experiences a problem, however, the wax can be removed, thus eliminating any sound blockage.

Infection

Infection occurring in the ear is called otitis, which simply means inflammation of the ear. Infection that occurs in the outer ear is called external otitis, and in the middle ear it is called otitis media. Both can result in a conductive hearing loss that is medically treatable.

External otitis. Infection in the outer ear is usually caused by bacteria on the skin of the ear canal. It may be very mild and produce only a slight itching, or it can cause swelling, drainage, and pain. Swimmer's ear occurs when the skin of the canal becomes infected, causing the canal to swell shut, and is a common example of external otitis. Although this condition produces a hearing loss by blocking sound, pain tends to be the overriding complaint. Other instances of external otitis are not usually as painful but can still block sound if there is sufficient swelling or drainage. Medicated eardrops are typically prescribed for external otitis. This treatment is usually successful to eliminate infection and reduce swelling so that sound can easily reach the eardrum once again.

Otitis media. This condition of otitis media exists when fluid or infection develops in the middle ear. As mentioned previously, the middle ear is supposed to be an air-filled space that allows easy movement of the eardrum and ossicles. Filling this part of the ear with fluid or infection literally puts a damper on the ability to hear. A malfunction of the Eustachian tube caused by a virus, by bacteria from an upper respiratory infection, by smoking, or by sinus problems can lead to otitis media. Instead of equalizing the pressure between the middle ear and outside world, the Eustachian tube fails to open, resulting in a vacuum within the middle ear. This vacuum pulls fluid from the surrounding tissue until the middle ear is filled. Not only does this fluid block sound, but it also creates an environment for bacterial growth.

Antibiotics are the primary treatment for otitis media. Most people are cured by following this therapy. If fluid remains in the middle ear, a physician can drain it in a procedure called a myringotomy. During this minor surgery the eardrum is numbed and then a small incision is made. Fluid within the middle ear is suctioned through this small hole.

After a few days the eardrum heals. If the fluid returns, a physician could repeat the myringotomy but this time insert a small tube in the myringotomy hole to aerate the middle ear. This pressure equalization tube would remain in the eardrum for about six to twelve months, allowing any blockage in the Eustachian tube to resolve. Almost all instances of otitis media and the resulting hearing losses can be cured.

Perforated Eardrum

A perforated or burst eardrum has a number of causes. A middle ear infection expanding until the pressure bursts through the eardrum is one common cause. Pressure from underwater diving, trauma from a slap on the ear, and accidents with cotton swabs are a few other examples. Small perforations usually heal by themselves within a few days. Larger perforations or repeated perforations are less likely to heal. Traumatic tears and those caused by an eardrum bursting can be extremely painful, producing a shooting pain or a searing sensation. Longstanding perforations can be painless or produce only a dull feeling. The amount of pain cannot be predicted by the size of the hole. The degree to which hearing is affected varies, depending on the size, shape, and location of the tear. A small hole usually has a negligible effect on hearing. A large hole is likely to have a larger impact because less sound is absorbed. The shape and placement of a perforation matter because they can affect how well the eardrum vibrates as a unit.

Eardrums that do not heal on their own can be repaired surgically. The simplest and least invasive approach is for a physician to apply a paper patch to the hole. The paper serves as a template, making it easier for the eardrum to heal. In cases of a traumatic perforation with no other pathology, a healing rate as high as 92 percent has been reported (Camnitz and Bost 1985). The success rate of this procedure decreases, however, when used on chronic perforations. In this situation the reported closure rate is 63.2 percent, 43.5 percent, and 12.5 percent for small, medium, and large perforations (Golz et al. 2003). Because of this decreasing success rate, paper patching is only appropriate in select cases.

A tympanoplasty is the procedure required to repair more serious tears. In this procedure, a vein or tissue graft is added beneath or over top of the eardrum remnants, with a closure rate of about 90 percent (Rizer 1997a, 1997b). A small perforation that does not heal on its own or after patching can also be repaired by tympanoplasty. If one attempt to close a perforation fails, a second surgery can still be successful. If it is not, water should be kept out of the ear. An intact eardrum serves as a barrier blocking bacteria, wax, and debris from entering the middle ear. Repairing a torn eardrum restores this protection.

Note that surgical success is often measured by closure of the perforation and not necessarily by hearing improvement. A reconstructed eardrum does not always work as efficiently as a healthy original. In a review of over seven hundred patients with tympanoplasties, about 55 percent were found to have no remaining conductive hearing loss after surgery. About 85 percent had an air–bone gap of 10 dB or less, and 90 percent had an air–bone gap of 15 dB or less (Rizer 1997b). One physician I know sometimes explains to a patient that he can make a good eardrum but that he cannot not make it as good as God. This sentiment honestly sums up what can be done with eardrum repair. Later chapters explain what can be done to improve hearing if surgery doesn't work.

Ossicular Damage

Infection and trauma often damage more than the eardrum. The bones in the middle ear may also be affected. They can be displaced or broken by trauma or eaten away by longstanding infection. Surgical treatments for ossicular problems vary greatly, depending on the type and extent of damage. Repositioning of existing structures or a prosthetic replacement may be necessary. Surgical reconstruction or replacement of the ossicles is called ossiculoplasty. Significant hearing improvements can result from surgery, but frequently there remains a difference between the hearing effectiveness of a normal and a reconstructed middle ear. In other words, ossicular replacements do not reproduce the lever action of the ossicles. The prosthesis may transfer sound well, but it does not have the sound-amplifying effect produced by the normal interplay of the ear bones. Ossiculoplasty is usually considered surgically successful if air conduction thresholds are brought to within 20 dB of bone conduction thresholds.

Cholesteatoma

A cholesteatoma is a benign skin growth within the middle ear. Most frequently, cholesteatoma occurs when there is a history of eardrum perforation or Eustachian tube dysfunction. When an eardrum tears, the outer layer of the eardrum may try to grow into the middle ear. This unwanted skin, along with the cells that are normally sloughed off, accumulates in the middle ear and becomes infected. In the case of Eustachian tube dysfunction, a negative pressure develops in the middle ear, causing an inward pull on the eardrum. A small portion of the eardrum may weaken and be sucked into the middle ear to form a pocket. Dead skin cells then accumulate within this pocket and become infected.

Drainage and odor are often the first signs of a cholesteatoma. Left untreated, it can erode the ossicles and ultimately lead to meningitis. The body of the cholesteatoma may not at first impede sound transmission, but hearing becomes affected over time.

A cholesteatoma is treated through surgery. The abnormal skin growth, infection, and damaged structures must all be removed. Although antibiotics may temporarily eliminate the infection, it will quickly return as long as the cholesteatoma remains. The chosen surgical procedure depends on the extent of damage and the physician's clinical judgment. A small cholesteatoma that has done little damage may be removed during a single surgery. In more severe cases, a series of surgeries, known as staging, is performed. One year after the original surgery, the ear is again opened to check for the recurrence of cholesteatoma. If there is regrowth, it is again removed. In severe cases the middle ear may not be reconstructed until the physician confirms that the cholesteatoma has not returned. Three or four surgeries are sometimes required to completely eradicate a cholesteatoma. Once this process is complete, a clinically successful hearing result (conductive hearing loss of 20 dB or less) can be obtained in about two-thirds of the cases (Schuring and Lippy 1985; Schuring et al. 1990).

Otosclerosis

Otosclerosis is a hereditary ear disease that can produce a conductive, mixed, or sensorineural hearing loss. This progressive disease most often starts during young adulthood but sometimes occurs in childhood or old age. Otosclerosis can affect one or both ears and is twice as common in women as in men.

Otosclerosis produces a spongy growth of bone over the stapes, locking this innermost ossicle in place. Up to a 60-dB conductive hearing loss can result from this fixation. Nerve damage can also occur with otosclerosis, although it is not entirely clear why.

The conductive hearing loss that results from otosclerosis can usually be corrected by a surgery called stapedectomy. Part or all of the stapes bone is removed during this surgical procedure. A vein graft is placed over this newly made opening between the middle and inner ear, and a prosthesis that connects to the incus is positioned against it. This reconstruction creates a movable ossicular chain that transmits sound efficiently. When an experienced surgeon performs this procedure, the size of the conductive hearing loss can be reduced to 10 dB or less in about 95 percent of the cases (Shea 1998; Rizer and Lippy 1993). What's more, stapedectomy can be just as effective when performed on people older than sixty-five (Lippy et al. 1996; Meyer and Lambert 2004).

A sensorineural hearing loss produced by otosclerosis, meaning that nerve cells are permanently damaged, is not correctable by stapedectomy. This means that in the case of a mixed hearing loss, the hearing can be improved by stapedectomy but some hearing loss will remain. Sensorineural hearing loss due to otosclerosis is sometimes treated medically with the nonprescription medicine sodium fluoride to keep the hearing from worsening (Shambaugh 1989). The prescription medication etidronate has also been suggested for this purpose (Brookler and Tanyeri 1997).

People suffering from otosclerosis are in good company, including the likes of Ludwig van Beethoven (Shearer 1990). Living over two hundred years ago and without the benefit of modern medicine, he went deaf. Tina, the baby boomer mentioned in chapter 1, is a more contemporary sufferer. You may recall that she had difficulty hearing in a number of situations and was especially unnerved by not being able to hear people behind her. Her audiogram showed an entirely conductive hearing loss and looked much like the one pictured in figure 3.4. She had a stapedectomy in one ear and then a stapedectomy in the other six months later. Today Tina has normal hearing and takes sodium fluoride to try to keep it that way.

If you require a stapedectomy, make sure an experienced practitioner performs the procedure because a successful outcome is linked to the doctor's level of experience (Hughes 1991; Sargent 2002). In one study, residents who performed stapedectomies had a 68 percent success rate compared with the 90 percent or greater success rate of experienced doctors (Backous et al. 1993). Research has also suggested a less than optimal success rate for surgeons who only occasionally perform the procedure (Puls 1997).

Autoimmune Inner Ear Disease

Autoimmune inner ear disease is one of the very few causes of sensorineural hearing loss that can be medically treated successfully. The progression of hearing loss can often be stopped or the hearing actually improved. Early diagnosis and treatment are key. Those individuals afflicted need to seek help early, and medical professionals need to be on watch for this exception to the rule that sensorineural hearing losses are permanent (Roland 2000). Autoimmune inner ear disease usually presents itself as a rapidly progressive hearing loss that occurs over a period of weeks or months. If this describes you, see an otologist or ENT physician now!

The cause of autoimmune disease is not well understood. A person's own immune system appears to damage the hearing nerves, resulting in sensorineural hearing loss. Laboratory tests such as the Western blot are often used diagnostically to look for the presence of certain antibodies in the blood that can indicate the disease (Garcia Callejo et al. 2003). Autoimmune inner ear disease is also diagnosed through a positive response to steroid therapy (Garcia Callejo et al. 2003; Ruckenstein 2004). If steroids are found to stabilize or improve hearing, the treatment may indicate an autoimmune disorder.

Ménière's Disease

Incapacitating vertigo, fluctuating hearing loss, roaring, and a sensation of fullness in the ear are all symptoms of Ménière's disease. The symptoms occur simultaneously in attacks that may last from a few hours to several days. The frequency of attacks is highly variable and may recur for five or ten years before the disease runs its course and the symptoms of dizziness lessen. Hearing thresholds usually improve between attacks, but there tends to be less hearing recovery over time. A moderate or severe sensorineural hearing loss often results from Ménière's disease.

The cause of Ménière's disease is thought to be a buildup of fluid that increases pressure in the inner ear and affects a person's sense of balance. Traditional medical treatment includes a low-salt diet and diuretics to try to limit the accumulation of fluid. A wide variety of other treatments is also available, including oral medications to minimize the severity of the dizziness, head exercises to strengthen and desensitize the balance system, gentamicin or dexamethasone injections to more directly treat the ear, and surgery to block dizzy signals from reaching the brain. The goal is to limit the frequency and severity of attacks and possibly reduce long-term hearing damage. Evaluating the effectiveness of competing treatments can be difficult because of the varying course of the disease. Whatever the treatment chosen, however, it should be started as early as possible to provide the greatest chance for a favorable outcome (Stahle 1984).

Sudden Hearing Loss

A sudden hearing loss is self-explanatory and can occur instantly or over the course of a few hours. If there is some question as to when a hearing loss occurred, it is probably not a sudden hearing loss. The sensorineural hearing loss may be partial or total. Although in rare cases it may occur in both ears, usually only one ear is affected. Sudden hearing loss is possibly the most frightening of hearing losses. If a person's hearing was normal yesterday and suddenly impaired today, what might tomorrow bring?

Sudden hearing loss is not a disease so much as a description of what has happened. The underlying etiology is not always well understood and may involve a variety of causes, including viral infection and vascular disease. Viral infections that damage the hearing nerves are contracted in many of the same ways as the common cold. A sudden hearing loss can also be caused by any interruption to the blood supply within or leading to the ear. Although some who have suffered sudden hearing losses will recover without treatment, the chance for hearing recovery is significantly improved through the use of oral steroids. For this treatment to be effective, however, it must be begun immediately or soon after the hearing loss (Chen et al. 2003; Slattery et al. 2005).

Acoustic Tumor

A small percentage of hearing loss is caused by a tumor damaging the nerve leading from the inner ear to the brain. This usually benign growth is called an acoustic neuroma or a vestibular schwannoma. It typically occurs in only one ear, although a rare hereditary condition known as neurofibromatosis causes it to occur bilaterally. A hearing loss most often develops gradually over months or years as the tumor grows. Hearing loss can sometimes occur suddenly. Therefore, it's important to suspect a tumor whenever there is a sudden hearing loss. Aside from unilateral hearing loss, other early signs of an acoustic tumor include dizziness, unilateral ringing or roaring in the ear (tinnitus), or a sense of pressure or fullness in the affected ear. The definitive test used to rule out or confirm an acoustic tumor is magnetic resonance imaging (MRI).

The traditional treatment for an acoustic tumor is surgical removal. A newer and less invasive treatment option is gamma knife radiosurgery. Although neither surgical removal nor radiation therapy will improve hearing that was damaged by an acoustic tumor, these procedures can sometimes make it possible for a person to preserve the hearing that remains. The prospect of a favorable result has improved in recent years as a result of the increased availability and use of MRI testing. This technology has resulted in tumors being detected earlier, when they are smaller and have done less damage (Stangerup et al. 2004).

Surmountable Hearing Loss

Although some hearing losses can be corrected or improved medically, the majority are sensorineural losses that cannot be reversed, making prevention especially important. Although these hearing losses are not medically correctable, they are usually surmountable.

Aside from noise-induced hearing loss, other recognized causes of permanent hearing loss include aging, heredity, and unknown etiology. Each of these problems is discussed in turn.

Aging

The medical term for hearing losses associated with aging is *presbycusis*, something of a catchall designation that throws together the many degenerative changes that cause sensorineural hearing loss with age. Hair cell death or dysfunction, reduced fluid movement resulting from a stiffening of the structures within the inner ear, and reduced ability of the nerves to create or transmit an electrical signal in response to sound are a few examples. Most hearing losses associated with age are bilateral and worsen gradually over many years. Not surprisingly, hearing thresholds and the rate of hearing change vary widely from person to person. Word understanding ability also varies. Men are more likely than women to have worse hearing as they age.

There is a tendency for people to dismiss age-related hearing loss as unavoidable. The underlying if unstated assumption here is that older people should be willing to settle for less. People say things like "My hearing isn't really so bad for my age" or "What do you expect when you're sixty-five?" but these statements do not alleviate communication problems and the social mishaps caused by the handicap, nor do they prevent the outside world from judging someone with such a loss negatively.

Heredity

Heredity is another cause for sensorineural hearing loss. A small percentage of people have a hereditary hearing loss at birth or one that develops in youth. Others may have a hereditary predisposition to hearing loss that only appears in middle age, late middle age, or old age. Those afflicted find their hearing thresholds or word understanding deteriorating faster than that of their peers, and without any obvious infection, disease, or pathology. The hearing nerves simply appear to be wearing out. An examination of family history often shows that someone suffering this condition has one or more family members with a similar unexplained deterioration.

Unknown

The medical term for a hearing loss of unknown etiology is *idiopathic*. Although professionals are able to identify the part of the ear affected, sensorineural hearing losses are often deemed idiopathic when there is no obvious cause or there are multiple possibilities such as heredity, noise exposure, or ototoxicity and it is not possible to differentiate between them. Interestingly, an idiopathic diagnosis in a younger person is often attributed to presbycusis in someone older. Even if there is no conclusive cause for an idiopathic loss, the location, severity, and pattern of hearing loss are known.

Compensating for Sensorineural Hearing Loss

Although the diagnosis of a permanent sensorineural hearing loss, as caused by noise exposure, heredity, or unknown causes, may seem like an insurmountable obstacle, there is still much that can be done to compensate for this kind of loss. Most people with sensorineural hearing loss can be helped with hearing aids, regardless of whether the cause is unknown or the result of noise exposure, aging, or heredity. Other assistive devices can also be tremendously helpful in listening situations that are found to be the most problematic. Options exist today that were not available a few years ago, and ongoing research offers the promise of additional advances, including the hope of a future cure.

Starting with hearing aids, the next few chapters examine the options and possibilities for coping with a hearing loss that cannot be medically corrected.

5 Hearing Aid Basics

The first electric hearing aids, made more than one hundred years ago, were based on the technology of the newly invented telephone. Most were the size of a small suitcase and encased in wood. A person had to wear a set of headphones or hold an earphone up to the ear in order to listen. Although these hearing aids were not small, discreet, or easily portable by today's standards, they were revolutionary for their time.

Hearing aids have improved dramatically from their early beginnings. The carbon amplifier adapted from the telephone was replaced by the vacuum tube, then by the transistor, and finally by the integrated circuit. Each advance in technology was accompanied by an increase in performance and a decrease in size. Today, there are very few hearing losses that cannot be helped with hearing aids.

This chapter explains hearing aid options and how to choose the style that will best work for a particular loss. Beyond the choice of circuit are add-ons such as a telecoil, which can make an aid easier to use with a telephone, or directional microphones, which offer hearing advantages in noise. I also discuss the hearing aid buyer's rights as a consumer and the question of whether to purchase one or two hearing aids.

Hearing Aid Styles

Hearing aids come in a variety of shapes and sizes and are categorized under several general styles. The most common of these as well as the key features of each are shown in figures 5.1 and 5.2. All of the hearing aids in figure 5.1 are custom-made to fit an individual ear. The earmold on the hearing aid in figure 5.2 is also custom-made for an individual ear. Because of this customization, the exact size and

Concha

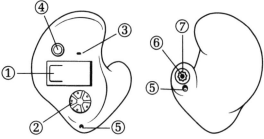

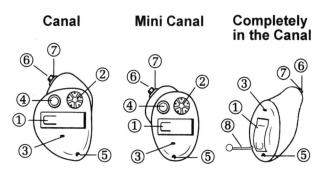

Canal   **Mini Canal**   **Completely in the Canal**

Figure 5.1. Sizes and landmarks of in-the-ear hearing aids. Landmarks: 1, battery door; 2, volume control; 3, microphone opening; 4, telecoil switch; 5, air vent; 6, sound outlet; 7, wax guard; 8, removal string. Photograph courtesy of Oticon Inc.

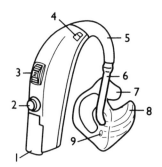

Figure 5.2. Landmarks of a behind-the-ear hearing aid with earmold. Landmarks: 1, battery door; 2, telecoil switch; 3, volume control; 4, microphone opening; 5, ear hook; 6, plastic tubing; 7, earmold; 8, sound outlet; 9, air vent. Photograph courtesy of Oticon Inc.

shape of a particular hearing aid style or earmold will vary from person to person.

Although there are some advantages to one hearing aid style over another, there is not usually a difference in quality between styles, just a better fit for each individual based on type of hearing loss, ear structure, and lifestyle. As a rule, larger hearing losses require the use of a larger hearing aid to allow more room for circuitry, a larger battery, and greater surface contact between the hearing aid and ear canal, ensuring that the amplified sound stays in the ear. The size and shape of an ear can also necessitate the use of one style over another. A very small ear may have insufficient space for an aid to fit entirely within the canal. A straight funnel-shaped canal may not provide enough retention to keep some hearing aid styles in place. Cosmetic concerns are often a big factor in selecting the style of hearing aid. There are obviously significant differences between styles in this regard. Care must be taken, however, to ensure that the choice of a small hearing aid that is cosmetically preferable is not made at the expense of hearing performance. Some hearing aid styles are inappropriate for some hearing losses.

The common styles of hearing aids shown in figures 5.1 and 5.2 are discussed in turn, as are some less common and specialized styles that are not shown.

Completely-in-the-Canal Hearing Aid

The completely-in-the-canal (CIC) hearing aid is the smallest style of hearing aid. As such, it is the least visible and is cosmetically preferable to larger styles. The entire aid fits within the ear canal, with the outermost edge slightly recessed from the canal opening. Because this placement makes it difficult to get a hold of the aid, a clear removal string is attached. A CIC aid works well with a mild hearing loss and is often recommended for moderate losses. More severe losses are typically considered beyond the fitting range of this style. An advantage of this aid aside from cosmetics is that the recessed placement usually makes a CIC aid useable with a telephone or headphone, or with a hat or scarf that is covering the ear. Some other hearing aids may whistle in these conditions. On the down side, the deep placement of a CIC aid, reaching into the bony portion of the ear canal, can make it less comfortable than other styles that do not go as deep. Battery life can be short because only the smallest button cell hearing aid battery (size 10) can be used. The small size may also limit the number of added options that can physically fit into this style of aid.

Mini Canal Hearing Aid

Although slightly larger than a CIC aid, a mini canal aid is still very discreet. A removal string may or may not be included, depending on the manufacturer and the anticipated difficulty of removal. The slightly larger size usually allows room for at least one user-adjustable control, such as a volume control, on the faceplate of the hearing aid. There is not generally room for this on a CIC aid, and even if there were, the placement of the aid would make it extremely difficult to adjust. A mini canal hearing aid can be used to compensate for about the same range of hearing loss as a CIC aid. Mini canal aids typically use the same small battery as CIC aids.

Canal Hearing Aid

A canal aid sits in the outer cartilaginous portion of the ear canal. This placement tends to make it more comfortable to wear than a deeper-fitting CIC aid. Although larger than CIC and mini canal aids, canal aids are not unsightly and often go unnoticed. When facing a hearing aid wearer, the small bump in front of the ear canal (the tragus) usually hides a canal aid from view, and the auricle hides the aid when viewed from the back. It can only be seen when viewed from the side. Canal aids do not usually require a removal string but usually do require a slightly larger battery (size 312) than a CIC or mini canal aid. This can supply more power or provide greater battery life. The increased shell size also allows more room for circuitry or added options. A canal aid is, as a rule, the smallest style that can begin to accommodate some of the larger hearing aid options such as a tele-coil or directional microphones (both discussed later). The ideal fitting range for a canal aid is mild to moderate losses.

Half-Shell Hearing Aid

A half-shell aid is in many ways like a canal aid except that it protrudes slightly farther out of the ear canal and fills up the lower half of the bowl-shaped portion of the ear. Aside from providing more space for circuitry, the increased shell size makes a more secure fit. Talking, chewing, yawning, and some other jaw movements can stretch the ear canal and occasionally loosen some of the smaller canal aids. A half-shell style fills the bottom portion of the ear, locking the hearing aid in place. This style is ideal for mild and moderate hearing losses and can sometimes be used with a more severe loss. It is also known as a half-concha aid.

Full-Shell Hearing Aid

The largest of the in-the-ear styles is the full-shell hearing aid, also known as a conch or in-the-ear (ITE) aid. The battery (size 13) is one size larger than the type used in a canal or half-shell aid, and two sizes larger than that used in a mini canal or CIC aid. This larger aid is most often used with moderate or severe hearing losses and provides greater surface contact with the ear, which helps to keep the sound in the ear where it belongs. The larger size of a full-shell aid also makes it the best choice for people with vision or dexterity problems. Any option that is available in the smaller hearing aid styles is also available in a full-shell aid. In fact, multiple features can be built into a full-shell style, while on smaller aids it is often necessary to pick and choose between them.

Behind-the-Ear Hearing Aid

Shown in figure 5.2, a behind-the-ear (BTE) hearing aid has two parts. The body houses the electronics and battery and is worn behind the ear. A clear tube attaches the body of the aid to a custom-fitted earmold. This arrangement may at first seem awkward, but it is very functional. The aid's circuitry is capable of providing a lot of power, and the earmold keeps sound in the ear as well or better than a full-shell aid. A BTE aid can also be quite acceptable cosmetically. A person's hair is frequently able to hide the body of the aid. If the earmold portion is made from a clear material, it can be less noticeable than a full or half-shell hearing aid. Behind-the-ear hearing aids are typically used with moderate, severe, or profound hearing losses. To minimize size, most BTE hearing aids use the same size 13 battery as a full-shell aid. When a great deal of power is required, as in the case of a severe or profound loss, a larger aid that holds a bigger battery (size 675) is used. Although there is a widespread perception that BTE aids are unsophisticated and old-fashioned, this view is unwarranted. Behind-the-ear hearing aids perform as well and sometimes better than smaller in-the-ear styles.

Eyeglass Hearing Aid

The eyeglass hearing aid is very similar in style to a BTE aid. Rather than being housed in a separate behind-the-ear unit, however, the works are integrated into the eyeglass frame. The earmold and tubing are identical to that used with a BTE, except that the tubing is connected to the temple portion of the eyeglass frame rather than to the BTE ear hook. Eyeglass hearing aids were popular when large plastic frames were in fashion. This older frame-style easily housed the hearing aid electronics and battery. Eyeglass hearing aids are rare now that wire and smaller plastic frames are in vogue.

Body Hearing Aid

The body hearing aid is the largest and most powerful style of hearing aid. The electronics and battery(s) are enclosed in a hard case that is about the size and shape of a pack of cigarettes. Some models are smaller, but any reduction in size is limited by the size of the AAA or AA batteries that power it. This device can sit in a pocket, be clipped to a belt, or placed in similar locations. A wire extends from the body of the aid to an earpiece or, with the use of a Y-cord, to two earpieces. Body-worn hearing aids have largely been replaced by BTE hearing aids. Aside from the cosmetic disadvantage, body-worn hearing aids have a tendency to pick up and amplify a number of unwanted sounds, such as stomach noises or clothing rubbing against the microphone. There are a few people with profound hearing loss who do better with a body aid than with any other style, but this is now the exception rather than the rule.

Contralateral Routing-of-Signal Hearing Aid

The contralateral routing-of-signal (CROS) style of hearing aid is designed for a person with normal hearing in one ear and no usable hearing in the opposite ear. Although this kind of loss may not pose a problem when a person is listening to someone situated in front or on the hearing-impaired person's better hearing side, it is a problem when trying to listen to someone on the nonhearing side. The bad ear can't hear, and the head is in the way of the good ear. Sound that does reach the good ear is greatly reduced in volume and therefore less audible. This reduction in volume is known as the *head shadow* effect. Unlike other hearing aids, a CROS aid does not send sound to the impaired ear. Instead, sound is picked up by a special aid worn on the nonhearing ear and transmitted through a wire or through radio waves to an aid worn in the good ear. It effectively keeps the head from getting in the way of the good ear, thereby eliminating any loss of sound.

Closely related to a CROS aid is a bilateral contralateral routing-of-signal (BICROS) hearing aid. This aid is designed for a person with some hearing loss in one ear and a total hearing loss in the other. Rather than merely transferring sound to the better ear, the hearing aid also provides amplification to this ear. CROS and BI-CROS aids are made in full-shell and behind-the-ear styles.

Noncustom Hearing Aids

All of the hearing aids that have been discussed up to this point are custom-made for an individual ear, which helps to ensure the best performance and most comfortable fit. In a different category are noncustom hearing aids. Here the manufacturer's approach is to make a one-size-fits-all or one-size-fits-most hearing aid that can be inexpensively mass-produced. Most are intended for an "average" canal shape and are designed to compensate for a high-frequency hearing loss since this configuration is most common. The disposable hearing aids that have been advertised on television from time to time are an example of a noncustom aid. The mail-order hearing aids featured in the back of numerous magazines are another example. Whether disposable or mail-order, a noncustom hearing aid can work well for some people, or it can instead fall out of a large ear, hurt a tiny ear, or compensate poorly for some types of hearing loss. Most would agree that noncustom hearing aids are less than ideal, but their lower cost leads many people to try them.

Hearing Aid Circuits

More than their size and shape, the electronics of a hearing aid matters. It is self-defeating to select a hearing aid solely on the basis of style without accounting for an appropriate circuit. For example, a person might insist on buying a CIC aid with the least expensive circuitry available. This is problematic because there is not usually room for a volume control, program button, or other adjustable controls, so the aid should include more advanced electronics to adjust to different listening situations. Therefore, selecting a circuit that cannot make these adjustments can be a prescription for failure. On the other hand, a fairly basic circuit may work well for a person who has relatively easy listening demands, especially if user-adjustable controls are included that allow the wearer to make adjustments that the electronics do not make.

A basic understanding of the available technology can help you select a hearing aid circuit that will work best with your hearing loss, listening needs, and hearing aid style. Hearing aid electronics have generally been categorized into three basic types: analog, programmable, and digital. A brief overview of each is provided here.

Analog

Analog is the technology that was traditionally—and often still is—used in radio, television, and home stereo. Analog devices process sound as an electrical voltage. Although this method of processing has been successful for many years, it has recently been given an unearned reputation for inaccurate sound reproduction. The shortcoming of analog technology is not sound quality but flexibility. Many analog devices are capable of processing sound with a level of distortion that is well below what is detectable by the human ear. Analog technology is problematic because it allows for only limited modification of sound. In hearing aid applications whose goal is to modify and then amplify the sound balance to best compensate for an individual hearing loss, this is a big limitation.

Early analog hearing aids amplified sound in a linear manner. All sound at a particular pitch was amplified the same amount, regardless of baseline loudness. This meant that if the aid was turned up loud enough to hear soft sounds, then loud sounds were increased to an uncomfortable level. If the aid was turned down so that the loud sounds were comfortable, then soft sounds were inaudible. This dilemma left the wearer fiddling with the volume control in search of the best compromise between hearing and comfort. A setting was later added that limited the maximum power output (MPO), but sounds that started out loud or moderately loud were still amplified at a level that proved overbearing to the user.

An amplification strategy called wide dynamic-range compression (WDRC) addressed some of the shortfalls of linear sound processing. This strategy varies the amount of amplification on the basis of input level. Soft sounds receive the most amplification. Progressively louder sounds receive less amplification. The goal was to make the widest possible range of sounds comfortably audible. This strategy offers clear advantages over linear amplification. It can make a soft whisper audible while keeping a loud shout from being uncomfortable. The problem is that the limited adjustability within analog hearing aids did not allow its optimal application. People with sensorineural hearing loss often have loudness intolerance at some pitches and not others. The WDRC in analog technology could not always be adjusted to account for these individual differences.

Programmable

In a programmable hearing aid, a computer-adjustable interface is added to an analog amplifier. This results in improved sound control over a basic analog aid. Adjustments for tone, loudness, or maximum power output made with a small screwdriver on the older version were largely a matter of trial and error. Adding a computer interface made it possible to better quantify any adjustment. The programmable display also made it easier to balance the sound between a pair of hearing aids or to return to a previous setting if the change wasn't suitable.

Being able to make subtle setting adjustments is crucial on WDRC hearing aids because if a WDRC aid is adjusted less than optimally, it can actually interfere with understanding. The process of giving greater amplification to soft sounds has the potential to obscure the sound of a person who is talking in a room with a lot of ambient noise. If the WDRC is set too aggressively, the wearer's ability to understand loud speech may be diminished because the aid provides little amplification to moderately loud sounds or actually reduces the volume. It may instead help to make people far away audible but not people who are close by. Any of these negative consequences can occur if the WDRC is not adjusted to an individual's hearing loss and listening environment. The improved sound control in programmable hearing aids increases the chance that the WDRC will be set appropriately.

Programmable hearing aids also make possible the option of multiple programs. One program can be set for listening in quiet environments, another for noisy environments, and a third for listening to music. A small push button on the face of the hearing aid allows the user to switch between programs as needed.

Digital

Digital hearing aids process sound as a series of numbers. The advantage to this form of processing is that sound can be modified in almost an infinite number of ways by simply changing a number here or there. The computer interface used with programmable analog hearing aids cannot provide the level of control that is possible with fully digital aids.

Digital hearing aids are increasingly becoming the model of choice. In 2000, about 25 percent of the purchased hearing aids were digital. By 2004, over 75 percent were digital (Strom 2004). This trend will likely continue until analog and programmable aids are mentioned only as a historical footnote in audiology textbooks.

Digital hearing aids are more and more being divided into entry-level, midlevel, and high-end categories. Minimizing cost tends to be the prime consideration in the entry-level category. Although these hearing aids work well and offer a limited number of features, they often perform much like their analog and programmable predecessors.

Midlevel digital aids are more adjustable than entry-level digitals. They separate the frequency range into several channels or bands that can be individually controlled. This can be a big advantage over single-channel analog and basic programmable and digital aids that control pitch, loudness, and compression less effectively. Midlevel digital aids may also include a wide array of features, including some basic form of background noise reduction.

High-end digitals can offer ten or more individually adjustable frequency bands. The many narrow bands in high-end hearing aids make it possible for hearing aid professionals to fine-tune the aids for individual listening needs or aggravations while minimizing any unwanted effect on other sounds. A computer programmer who is bothered by the sound of computer fans may be able to minimize this aggravation by a minor adjustment within one narrow hearing aid band. A farmer who is bothered by the sound of chickens might find relief by regulating a different band. The latest in noise cancellation, directional microphones, and other leading-edge features to be discussed shortly are likely to be available or included with high-end digitals.

Hearing Aid Options

Choosing the most appropriate hearing aid add-ons can be as or more important than selecting a style and circuit. The extra features chosen depend on listening needs and lifestyle rather than the amount of hearing loss. This section discusses a number of common hearing aid options and the situations in which they may be most helpful.

Multiple Programs

The option of having multiple programs for use in different situations is available on many programmable and digital hearing aids. A small push button on the hearing aid faceplate lets a user select between programs at will. This feature increases the flexibility of a hearing aid.

Hearing aids are programmed to emphasize speech sounds. The balance of pitches that is best for understanding speech, however, is not always the ideal setting for listening to music, nature, or other sounds. Music, for example, requires the faithful reproduction of sound. A hearing aid emphasizing speech will cut off the extreme low and high frequencies and may alter the balance of sounds that remain, leading to a distortion in the music. Furthermore, a program designed for listening to speech in a quiet room may not be optimal for listening to speech in a noisy crowd. Even types of noise make a difference. A truck driver's greatest concern may be eliminating road noise, whereas a waiter is more likely to be concerned about background speech and reverberation. A program that deals well with one noise source many not function well in the presence of another.

Directional Microphones

The standard hearing aid microphone is omnidirectional, amplifying sound from multiple directions. An omnidirectional microphone makes a speaker audible whether he or she is in front, behind, or on the side of a listener. The microphone's function allows a person to hear everything, but there are times when this panoramic sound processing can interfere with hearing. For example, when at a restaurant, a hearing aid user might hear the conversation of diners two tables away as loudly as that of the person at the table with her. A restaurant full of people becomes a jumble of voices. Welcome to the world of omnidirectional microphones.

The alternative to this menagerie of noise is to use a directional microphone that can allow the wearer to focus on sound coming from only one area. A directional microphone does not block surrounding sounds but amplifies them less than sounds coming from the front. In our restaurant example, this device would limit the overall jumble of voices for the listener yet still make it possible to hear someone at his or her table. Directional microphones can make a big difference when trying to hear in loud settings. Unfortunately, this option is often overlooked during the hearing aid buying process.

Although there are many circumstances in which directional microphones are beneficial, they are not a good full-time solution. Hearing from all directions is preferable to targeted hearing when driving, riding a bike, taking a walk, or crossing the street. Fortunately, it is not necessary to choose between directional and omnidirectional microphones since most hearing aids have room for both, and the wearer can select either as needed.

Telecoil

The telecoil, a feature designed to assist with telephone conversations, uses a method called magnetic induction to process the electromagnetic energy produced by the phone. Fluctuations in the telephone earpiece's magnetic field induce a voltage across the wires within the telecoil that is then processed as sound. Although this may seem like a lot of fuss since it is standard that hearing aids come with a microphone that can process sound, there are a number of reasons that a telecoil can be worthwhile.

First, hearing aids have a tendency to whistle if they are covered. No matter how well a hearing aid is fitted to an ear, often a little sound manages to work its way around the aid and escape the ear. In normal use this is not a problem. If an aid is covered, however, this sound is directed into the hearing aid microphone to be amplified again. This starts a feedback cycle in which sound is amplified again and again until all an aid can do is whistle at its maximum loudness. It is possible to prevent this cycle by holding the phone slightly away from the hearing aid, but this can be awkward and can reduce the ability to hear. A telecoil eliminates this problem because the microphone is turned off and any sound escaping the ear is ignored because the aid is detecting electromagnetic energy instead.

A telecoil is also advantageous because it blocks outside sounds during phone conversations. Because the microphone is turned off, only the person speaking on the telephone is heard. This can be a big help when conducting a conversation over the phone in noisy settings.

More than improving telephone communication, a telecoil also allows for improved listening in other venues. Theaters, lecture halls, tourist attractions, and many other public and private places are equipped to provide hearing assistance through a telecoil.

A small push button on the hearing aid faceplate is typically used to toggle between the microphone and telecoil. In hearing aids with multiple options such as a directional microphone and a telecoil, a single switch may be used to select between them. More convenient than a manual switch is an automatic telecoil. This feature senses when the hearing aid is near a telephone or other strong electromagnetic source and automatically turns the telecoil on.

Volume Control

A volume control was essential for older hearing aids because they were not sophisticated enough to automatically adjust sounds to the best volume. Newer hearing aids do a much better job than older aids at keeping sound at an optimal hearing level. The need for a hearing aid user to adjust the volume manually is not as crucial. This does not mean, however, that a wearer never wants the flexibility of a manual control. A person might wish to hear an important conversation louder than the level presented by a hearing aid's programming. The individual might choose to lower the volume on an offensive conversation. Obviously, personal and situational factors frequently influence what a person would like to hear, and the inclusion of a volume control on some high-end hearing aids is an acknowledgment of this fact.

Remote Control

A remote control is another feature that can be purchased with a few high-end hearing aids. For small CIC hearing aids with no room for a user-adjustable control on the aid itself, a remote control may be the only way for a wearer to adjust the aid. On larger aids, a remote can eliminate the need for a clutter of small switches that may be hard to adjust. It can also make an aid easier to adjust for someone who has a problem with dexterity. Whereas some people do not like a remote because it costs extra and is an additional item to remember and carry, others find it to be a useful option.

Windscreen

A windscreen is a low-technology feature that is useful but not widely advertised. It is the functional equivalent of the foam ball with which television reporters cover their microphone to protect against wind noise. Some hearing aids come standard with a windscreen, a fine mesh that covers the hearing aid microphone opening. Others are designed with a microphone placement or opening that minimizes wind noise. A few hearing aids come with no standard accommodation to protect against wind. If the wearer likes to golf, fish, garden, walk, jog, hike, bike, or engage in other outdoor activities, minimizing wind noise should be a consideration.

Wax Guard

Earwax is perhaps the greatest nemesis of hearing aids. Physically inserting a hearing aid into the ear canal can scoop up any wax sitting in the canal. This sometimes results in an aid needing constant cleaning to prevent wax from blocking the sound opening. Even with diligent care, however, the wax may accumulate in hard-to-clean places, where it may even cause damage to the aid.

A number of hearing aid manufacturers have designed special guards to protect against wax. These usually consist of a small screen or barrier at the entrance of the sound opening. Some are semipermanent and can only be cleaned by a hearing aid professional. Others are disposable and can easily be changed by the user. Anyone with a history of wax buildup should regard this option as essential. Furthermore, selecting a hearing aid that is protected by a wax guard is a good idea for anyone since a buildup that would not cause any problem in an ear canal can cause problems for a hearing aid. A wax guard adds little or no cost when purchasing a hearing aid and may prevent a great deal of aggravation later.

Other Hearing Aid Basics

Of the few hearing aid issues still to be discussed, one of the biggest is whether to purchase one hearing aid or two. I also review the questions to ask and factors to consider when purchasing hearing aids.

One Hearing Aid versus Two

One of the most frequent questions regarding hearing aid use is whether two hearing aids are necessary or whether one is sufficient. The short answer is that one hearing aid is usually better than none, but two are best. Exceptions to this rule include a person with a hearing loss in only one ear or a loss in one ear that is so severe as to be unaidable. Since most hearing losses occur bilaterally, however, the most favorable outcome is likely to be obtained by restoring sound to both ears.

The most obvious benefit of improved amplification in both ears is the ability to localize sound. Although a person may hear with one hearing aid, some clairvoyance may be required to determine the direction of the sound. If the wearer does not have improved hearing in both ears, the sound will seem to be coming from the side that has the aid, which will be a problem unless the wearer can see the source of the sound. More than an inconvenience, it is also a safety issue. One need only consider the necessity of identifying the direction of a honking horn while driving to realize the importance of the ability to locate a sound source.

It is harder to hear in noisy environments without the assistance of two hearing aids. The brain compares what one ear hears versus the other to sort things out in difficult listening environments. Subtle loudness and timing differences among sounds reaching the ears are key to helping the brain separate one voice from a muddle of sound. Without these cues, an individual voice may remain part of the muddle. The advantage of binaural processing for understanding in noise has long been documented (Wright and Carhart 1960; Carhart 1965; Dermody and Byrne 1975).

Remember that in the case of single-sided deafness, a person's head blocks sound from reaching the good ear. This head shadow effect additionally applies when only one hearing aid is worn when two are needed. A single aid may help when sound is coming from the front or side, but an aid will be of limited benefit for hearing sound on the opposite side. With the exception of single-sided deafness, wearing two hearing aids usually makes it possible to hear sound regardless of side.

In 1984 Silman and his colleagues discovered another argument favoring binaural hearing aids. They found that some people who wear only one hearing aid experience a worsening of word understanding ability in the unaided ear. Hearing thresholds remain unaffected. These findings were confirmed by later studies (Gelfand et al. 1989; Emmer 1990; Burkey and Arkis 1993). The end result is that after years of monaural hearing aid use, an unaided ear that may have started out providing some help becomes less helpful over time. Adding a hearing aid to the previously unaided ear has been found to reverse the word understanding deterioration in some but not all cases (Silverman and Emmer 1993; Arkis and Burkey 1994; Gelfand 1995). This risk does not apply if the unaided ear has perfect hearing.

Making a Hearing Aid Choice

Selecting a particular brand of hearing aid is one of the first choices to be made during the purchasing process. A short alphabetical list of some of the major hearing aid brands is shown in box 5.1. Some

---

Box 5.1. Twelve established hearing aid manufacturers

Beltone	Oticon	Sonic Innovations
GN ReSound	Phonak	Starkey
Magnatone	Rexton	Unitron
Miracle Ear	Siemens	Widex

---

companies such as Beltone and Miracle Ear are well known because they advertise extensively to the public. These well-publicized companies are not, however, the only quality manufacturers of hearing aids. A professional may recommend hearing aids from one of the lesser-advertised companies listed here or from a smaller company he or she knows to be good. Although brand is a definite consideration in the purchase of hearing aids, it should probably not be the first consideration.

A better starting point is the style of hearing aid. The first question to ask a hearing aid professional is: What style of hearing aid is appropriate for my hearing loss? Once you have this information, do not insist on a style that is not appropriate for you. Your second task is to select the hearing aid circuit and special features that best meet your lifestyle and listening needs. A hearing aid professional can help you sort through these options. Once you know what you want in a hearing aid, then you can return to brand selection. Frequently, several good hearing aid companies can make hearing aids to meet your specific needs. An experienced hearing aid professional will know which combinations of features are available from which manufacturers.

Hearing Aid Prices

The average price of a hearing aid ranges from $900 to $3,000, depending on style, circuit, and brand (Strom 2005). A breakdown of average prices by style is shown in box 5.2 for economy, midlevel, and premium digital hearing aids. Basic add-ons such as a windscreen, wax guard, or telecoil are often included in the price. More expensive features such as a directional microphone that may add $150 to $200 to the cost of an economy hearing aid are often included in the price of a midlevel or high-end aid.

Box 5.2. Average prices for digital behind-the-ear (BTE), in-the-ear (ITE), canal, and completely-in-the-canal (CIC) hearing aids

	BTE	ITE	Canal	CIC
Economy aid	$1,428	$1,409	$1,514	$1,742
Midlevel aid	$1,968	$1,960	$2,050	$2,292
Premium aid	$2,509	$2,511	$2,587	$2,842

Source: Strom 2005.

Understanding the Purchasing Process

Custom hearing aids can be purchased from audiologists and hearing instrument specialists. The professional training and scope of practice for audiologists was discussed in chapter 4. In contrast to the formal education required to become an audiologist, hearing instrument specialists usually learn their trade on the job. They are, however, required to demonstrate competency before state licensure. Although hearing aids are also dispensed in otology and ENT offices, it is most often a staff audiologist who does the fitting in these settings and not the physician.

The fitting process begins with an audiologist or hearing instrument specialist making an impression of the ear so that a hearing aid can be formed to this exact shape. The procedure is painless and involves the placement of a small foam or cotton ball into the ear canal followed by a quick-hardening impression material. This cast, along with circuitry specifications, is then sent away to a hearing aid manufacturer. About two weeks later, the hearing aid is mailed from the manufacturer, and the audiologist or hearing instrument specialist programs it to an individual's specific needs. A little fine-tuning of the aid's programming may occur later, depending on feedback provided by the wearer.

Regardless of where in the United States hearing aids are purchased, the buyer has certain consumer rights. The most important of these is the guarantee that the hearing aids can be returned within a set period of time (usually thirty days) if the wearer is dissatisfied for any reason. If the hearing aids are returned, the purchase price is refunded minus an agreed-upon trial fee. The amount of this fee is included in the sales agreement and should not exceed 10 percent of the purchase price of the hearing aids. Knowing the buyer has this option can alleviate many concerns about purchasing an expensive but possibly ineffectual tool.

6   Satisfaction and Dissatisfaction with Hearing Aids

The last chapter presented hearing aids as a successful cutting-edge technology that for many years has improved the listening ability of those who wear them and in recent years has become far more effective. Unfortunately, however, many complain about hearing aids for both legitimate and misinformed reasons.

Ten of the most common hearing aid complaints are shown in box 6.1. There are many more. Fewer than 25 percent of persons with hearing loss who could be helped with hearing aids actually buy them (Kochkin 1993; Weinstein 1996) because of the perception that hearing aids are more trouble than they are worth.

Some of these perceptions come from trying to view hearing aids as a cure rather than as a way to compensate for a hearing loss. Although hearing aids can almost always improve a hearing-impaired person's ability to communicate, they do not restore normal hearing. No matter how much hearing aids may help, there is still a gap between normal hearing and hearing aid–enhanced hearing that leaves room for dissatisfaction.

Hearing well in noise with hearing aids can be a problem for several reasons. The first applies to everyone whether they are hearing impaired or not. Hearing in noise is more difficult than hearing in quiet. One sound can obscure other sounds, or noises can blend together to make individual sounds indistinguishable from one another. Wearing hearing aids is not a cure for these acoustic realities. Novice hearing-aid users have an additional problem that usually improves over time. They frequently complain about background noise being distracting or overwhelming because their hearing loss has made them accustomed to a quiet world. Reintroduction to an environment full of sound can be unsettling and take a long time to get used to.

Box 6.1. Ten common complaints about hearing aids

1. People who wear hearing aids still don't hear.
2. Hearing aids have poor sound quality.
3. Hearing aids don't work if there is background noise.
4. Hearing aids make background noise overwhelming.
5. People who buy hearing aids don't wear them.
6. Hearing aids buzz and whistle all the time.
7. Hearing aids are uncomfortable.
8. Hearing aids need constant maintenance.
9. Hearing aids are big and ugly.
10. People who wear hearing aids become dependent on them.

The gap between normal and hearing aid–enhanced hearing is most often evident when trying to understand speech. Sensorineural hearing loss not only affects hearing sensitivity but can also affect word understanding ability—especially in noisy settings. Hearing aids can make speech sounds audible, thereby improving the likelihood of understanding, but they cannot correct the underlying nerve damage that contributes to word understanding difficulties. Many hearing aid complaints originate here.

As explained previously, hearing aids are programmed to emphasize speech sounds, sometimes at the expense of perceived sound quality. Depending on the wearer's pattern of hearing loss, the hearing aid settings that provide the best word understanding can be quite different from the frequency balance that sounds closest to natural voices. This does not mean that voices will sound distorted—as though Darth Vader is talking. They may, however, sound like there is too much treble, base, or mid-frequency emphasis. The intentional choice to maximize speech understanding is often named as a fault. In addition, hearing aids are often faulted for sound quality issues caused by the sensorineural hearing loss and not the hearing aid itself. Sound distortions in the inner ear can occur with sensorineural hearing loss, and there is no way that hearing aids can correct this problem.

The often negative perception of hearing aids is partly a result of exaggeration. Although hearing aids can make a whistling noise called feedback if they are covered or do not fit an ear properly, feedback is rare if the aid is properly fitted. In addition, hearing aids do not feel uncomfortable or require constant maintenance, but they do need a minimum of care to work properly. Although some people who purchase hearing aids do not use them, over 90 percent of hearing aid owners *do* use them (Kochkin 2002).

Many people give cosmetic reasons for their opposition to wearing hearing aids, but their underlying objections often are based on issues surrounding fear of aging and dependence. In truth, today's hearing aids are much smaller and more cosmetically acceptable than in the past. The smallest CIC aids can be nearly invisible to the naked eye, yet people complain about them. Fears of aging, disability, and decline as well as taboos of our youth-oriented society can lead a person to avoid hearing aids because buying one may be viewed as an affirmation of aging.

Another common fear is that people who wear hearing aids become dependent on them. After all, it is well known that when you change to a higher-strength eyeglass prescription, your eyes become increasingly dependent on the lenses. Not so with hearing aids. Although hearing aids help a person to hear better, they do not diminish the underlying ability to hear. Hearing aids do, however, increase a person's expectation to hear. With this expectation, a person then uses and depends on his or her hearing aids more. Hearing aids are tools that can help a person maximize the chance to hear. Hearing itself is the real object of dependence.

Dissatisfaction with hearing aids does not mean they are not helpful. People may be annoyed that they have to rely on them, and this frustration is expressed in negative feelings toward hearing aids even when they provide tremendous benefit. When patients of mine say they dislike their hearing aids, I ask why they wear them. They usually reply, "Because I need them to hear." Although this response does not surprise me, it is surprising to an observer. Observers typically view hearing aid dissatisfaction as a confirmation that the aids provide no benefit. Clearly, this view is often not the case.

Hearing Aid Benefits

Hearing aid wearers who speak negatively of their aids may also overlook the benefits. Fortunately, there are ways to assess the pros and cons of hearing aids aside from asking a wearer's opinion of them. Comparing what a person hears with the use of hearing aids versus without can serve as one determination of hearing aid benefits. These benefits can also be assessed on the basis of their impact on quality of life: Do hearing aids eliminate or reduce the handicap imposed by hearing loss? Do they make it possible for a hearing-impaired person to accomplish more? The following discussion examines hearing aid benefits from each of these perspectives.

Improved Hearing Ability

Hearing aids have always improved a wearer's ability to hear to some degree. These days, technology has made the aids even better. Hearing aids are prescription fitted based on the amount of hearing loss. Until recently, most hearing aid prescriptions employed some variation on a half-gain formula that corrected for about one-half of a given hearing loss. For example, a 40-dB loss was improved to a 20-dB loss, and a 60-dB loss was improved to a 30-dB loss. This formula was a compromise between trying to make speech sounds audible without making them uncomfortably loud. Although this did not restore normal hearing, it did result in a quantifiable improvement.

With the advent of wide dynamic-range compression, prescriptive hearing aid formulas have become more complex. Two popular fitting methods include the desired sensation level input/output (DSL I/O) and National Acoustics Laboratories–nonlinear (NAL-NL1) procedures (Cornelisse et al. 1995; Byrne et al. 2001). In each of these formulas the amount of amplification varies as a function of two factors—hearing loss and initial sound level. Soft sounds are amplified more than moderate sounds; moderate sounds are amplified more than loud sounds. In this way, listening comfort and the ability to hear are considered by each formula, and users often report a higher satisfaction level. The NAL-NL1 formula additionally balances the perceived loudness between frequencies, which may help to produce a more natural sound balance. Some compromise between audibility and comfort is still required with DSL I/O and NAL-NL1, but formulas such as these better utilize today's hearing aid technology.

Repeating the hearing test with the use of a hearing aid is one objective way to determine whether or not an aid is performing its job. This aided testing is done in a similar manner to unaided testing, except that sounds are presented through speakers rather than headphones. Hearing sensitivity and word understanding ability can both be evaluated. The comparison of aided to unaided testing was used for years with linear hearing aids to confirm that the person with hearing difficulties was using the most appropriate settings. Although this testing method can be used with newer hearing aids to gain a general idea of performance, it can be inadequate for assessing the subtle sound manipulations that take place in digital signal processing and wide dynamic-range compression hearing aids.

Newer hearing aids are best evaluated electronically with a hearing aid analyzer. This device sends a variety of calibrated signals through a hearing aid and measures the output. It can accurately measure the amount of amplification, distortion, and sound compression provided by an aid. Hearing aid manufacturers routinely perform this test on new hearing aids to ensure that their many functions work properly. Hearing aid professionals also perform this test to confirm that the hearing aid programming is appropriate for an individual's hearing loss. A slight variation on this system (real-ear measurement) tests the output of an aid while it is in a person's ear by extending a thin tube alongside the hearing aid and into the ear canal. By measuring the sound level at the eardrum, this method shows not only the output of the hearing aid but also determines how the size, shape, and resonance of an individual's ear canal affect the sound. Real-ear measurement can confirm that the sound balance reaching the eardrum is appropriate for an individual's hearing loss. The test results also show which sounds will be audible to a hearing aid wearer.

Quality of Life

As discussed in previous chapters, hearing loss affects social functioning and work performance. Loneliness, isolation, reduced independence, and depression can result from poor hearing. The ability of hearing aids to help a person overcome these negative consequences confirms the benefits of using them.

Quality-of-life changes resulting from hearing aid use were studied at a Bureau of Veterans Affairs hospital (Mulrow et al. 1990). Researchers separated 194 consecutive hearing-impaired patients into two groups. The first group was fit with hearing aids, and the second group received no intervention. A battery of quality-of-life measures performed before and after the hearing aid fitting showed that the hearing aid group experienced significant quality-of-life improvements relative to the control group, including improved social and emotional function, better communication, higher cognitive function, and a lessening of depression. The researchers concluded that adverse quality-of-life effects resulting from hearing loss are reversible with hearing aids.

Later quality-of-life research reinforced the value of hearing aids. A study of more than a thousand elderly people showed that hearing aids improved the quality of life of the study group and may have even protected against cognitive impairment and disability (Cacciatore et al. 1999). A smaller study that included fifty adults also found improvement in social and emotional functioning with the wearing of hearing aids (Lamden et al. 1995). Furthermore, most quality-of-life improvements are sustained with continued hearing aid use. Researchers found this to be true for improvements in communication, depression, and social and emotional well-being (Mulrow et al. 1992). Interestingly, hearing aid use also improves the quality of life for relatives of the hearing impaired, partially because they experience a decline in aggravation from having to constantly repeat themselves and endure the higher volume of the television, radio, and other electronic devices that their loved one requires (Brooks et al. 2001; Stark and Hickson 2004). These studies illustrate that despite many complaints, there is no doubt that hearing aids can improve the life of the wearer and his or her family.

Hearing Aid Satisfaction

Learning what has helped others make the most of their hearing aid experiences can help a wearer to maximize his or her own satisfaction. Yet satisfaction is subjective, so a hearing outcome that is perceived as satisfactory by one person may not be by another. Satisfaction can be an elusive if not a moving target.

Comparison with Other Products

To gain some perspective on how satisfied hearing aid users are with their aids, psychologist Sergei Kochkin (2003b) compared how people felt about their hearing aids with their level of satisfaction with other products and services. For nonprogrammable hearing aids, that is, hearing aids that cannot be computer programmed to individual listening needs, he reported a satisfaction level of only 58 percent. This result was comparable to people's satisfaction with the Internal Revenue Service or gas and electric utilities. However, people with high-end hearing aids that included the most advantageous features such as multiple memories or background noise reduction were reported as having a satisfaction level of 81 percent, a score comparable to ratings of cars and consumer electronics. This was slightly better than the average rating for beer! Although it may be overly optimistic to claim that people would prefer hearing aids to beer, this study shows that the range of satisfaction experienced with hearing aids is comparable to that of other products and services.

Hearing Aid Benefit and Satisfaction

So what causes an increase in satisfaction with hearing aids? Kochkin (2003b) found a strong relationship between reduced hearing disability and improved hearing aid satisfaction. When perceived hearing disability was improved by 50 percent, overall hearing aid satisfaction was 72 percent. Satisfaction jumped to 95 percent when the perception of nearly perfect hearing was obtained. This means that selecting the hearing aids most suited for a particular hearing loss and listening needs will offer the wearer the greatest chance for satisfaction. The selection can best be made by using the recommendations of an audiologist or hearing instrument specialist.

Hearing Aid Size and Satisfaction

A 1994 study examining the impact of hearing aid style on likely purchasers shows how satisfaction can be influenced by hearing aid size (Kochkin 1994). Hearing-impaired subjects in this study were asked to view a series of color photographs of different hearing aid sizes and styles pictured in an ear. They were then asked to rate their likelihood of buying each style. Not surprisingly, small styles such as a CIC aid were greatly preferred over larger styles such as a BTE aid. People perceived the smaller hearing aids to be of better quality and predicted they would outperform larger hearing aids. But this is not usually the case. As Kochkin said: "Because innovative technology tends to be introduced into large hearing instruments first, this finding has serious implications for market acceptance of larger hearing instruments, regardless of their level of sophistication in signal processing." Let this be a warning to be open-minded about trying a larger hearing aid style if recommended by a professional and not to be fooled by its bulkier appearance. In the case of hearing aids, sleeker isn't always better.

Special Features and Satisfaction

Some features are accurately perceived as improving the hearing aid experience for many users. Wide dynamic-range compression (WDRC) is a perfect example. As previously explained, WDRC is a method of amplifying sound while controlling loudness. The goal is to make sound audible but not uncomfortable. A secondary goal is to preserve a sense of normal loudness growth so that sounds do not suddenly become loud or drop from audibility. WDRC is often identified as one of the factors responsible for making newer hearing aids preferable to older technology (Noffsinger et al. 2002; Larson et al. 2002). However, WDRC can also provide a noticeable benefit in older, nondigital hearing aid styles (Walden et al. 2000). Fortunately, most new hearing aids, whether analog, programmable, or digital, use some form of WDRC.

The option of multiple memories is another feature accurately associated with improved satisfaction. Obviously, a person who needs to hear in diverse listening conditions will do better with and prefer hearing aids that include separate settings for these different conditions. Findings from the National Acoustics Laboratory in Australia support this view (Keidser 1995). When subjects compared sixteen amplification schemes in fifteen different listening conditions, 84 percent of the subjects preferred different amplification schemes depending on the number of talkers, background noise, and so forth.

If you are considering add-on features for your hearing aid, a multiple memory button should be at the top of your list.

Directional microphones are another potential add-on designed to improve hearing in background noise, a frequent complaint of people with hearing loss and an even more frequent complaint of people who wear hearing aids. In chapter 5, I mentioned the option of incorporating a directional microphone into a hearing aid, thereby limiting surrounding sounds. In terms of benefit, directional amplification has been shown to improve speech understanding in many noisy environments. However, users do not overwhelmingly perceive this device as beneficial (Ricketts and Mueller 2000). Self-assessment measures have found directional microphones to be seen as positive, neutral, or negative depending on the specific listening situation (Ricketts et al. 2003). Increased satisfaction from being able to understand speech better from the front may be countered by not hearing as well from the back or sides. Don't disregard this feature, however; in chapter 8 I offer a solution to getting the most out of directional microphone technology.

Even a feature as simple as a volume control can affect hearing aid satisfaction. Older hearing aids almost always included a volume control because the circuitry was not sophisticated enough to keep sound at optimal or comfortable levels. With the advent of WDRC and programmable and digital hearing aids that should be "self-adjusting," volume controls became less common and were omitted from many hearing aid models. Addressing this trend, Kochkin (2003a) noted that "categorical removal of instrument controls, particularly volume controls . . . , has undoubtedly led to unnecessary frustration and anger among some consumer segments." A study of experienced hearing aid users reported that about three-fourths of the subjects preferred to have a volume control, even if they used it only occasionally (Surr et al. 2001). Even with digital hearing aids, a volume control remains a useful option that should not be considered old-fashioned.

User Factors That May Affect Satisfaction with Hearing Aids

Although much of the credit or blame related to satisfaction or dissatisfaction with hearing aids is attributed to the technology, it is not the only factor affecting satisfaction. User expectations almost certainly play a role. Someone with low expectations may be very pleased if hearing aids can provide even minimal benefit. Someone with higher expectations may be dissatisfied even if the hearing aids are of great help. One recurring theme found in surveys of new hearing aid users is that expectations frequently exceed what can actually be achieved with amplification (Schum 1999; Cox and Alexander 2000). Unfortunately, hearing aid advertising often compounds rather than corrects unrealistic expectations. Baby boomers with high expectations must recognize that even current technology has its limits.

A person's level of social activity has also been associated with hearing aid satisfaction. A study done in Cologne, Germany, found that people who are active socially report higher benefit and satisfaction for all listening conditions (Meister et al. 2004). This finding should not be surprising since increased communication demands result in a greater need for hearing aids. Still, caution is in order because research shows that hearing aid satisfaction cannot reliably be predicted based solely on perceived need (Schum 1999). However, a typical baby boomer with an active social life and career but who is currently hard of hearing can safely bet that hearing aids will improve his or her interactions.

It is not uncommon for hearing aid professionals to see a person with hearing loss who has been hauled into their office by a friend or relative. The person may deny any hearing problem but still purchase hearing aids under duress. Later the hearing aids go unworn or unappreciated. I have seen it happen many times. This is an extreme example of how acceptance of hearing loss can affect hearing aid outcome. In her 1969 book *On Death and Dying*, Elizabeth Kubler-Ross describes five stages a person passes through when faced with the prospect of dying, including denial, anger, bargaining, depression, and acceptance. Her premise that a person must come to accept the prospect of death before being able to deal effectively with it has gained wide acceptance. This idea has successfully been applied to other situations involving loss, including hearing loss, and it has been incorporated into hearing aid studies (Jerram and Purdy 2001). A person who does not accept his or her hearing loss is unlikely to accept hearing aids. A person who fully accepts the loss is likely to be more satisfied with hearing aids than a person who only partially acknowledges the problem.

Burt, one of the patients mentioned in chapter 1, exemplifies the problem of denial. He had a significant hearing loss that almost certainly could have been helped with hearing aids, but he denied the problem, instead blaming those around him for his listening difficulties. Had Burt somehow been convinced to buy hearing aids as his family would have preferred, it is unlikely that he would have worn them and even less likely that he would have been happy with them. He first had to accept his hearing loss.

Possible Tests to Predict Hearing Aid Satisfaction

Understanding in spite of background noise varies from person to person and has already been mentioned as a frequent problem affecting satisfaction with hearing aids. Therefore, it seems reasonable that evaluating a person's ability to understand speech during noise might be one way to predict hearing aid benefit and consequently satisfaction. If a person can understand clearly presented speech regardless of background noise, then he or she would likely do well, and be satisfied with, hearing aids. If the auditory system cannot separate speech from noise, then a person would be a less promising hearing aid candidate. Unfortunately, there does not appear to be a predictive relation between the speech-in-noise measures currently available and patients' reported hearing aid benefit (Cord et al. 2000). One study that did suggest a relationship noted that much of the perceived relation was likely attributable to other factors (Walden and Walden 2004).

A different approach in trying to predict hearing aid satisfaction focuses not on understanding in noise but rather on a person's tolerance for listening in noise. The idea is that those who have a greater willingness to listen in noise will do better with hearing aids. An acceptable noise level (ANL) is calculated in decibels and represents the difference between the most comfortable listening level for speech and the highest background noise level that is acceptable. People who accept background noise have smaller ANLs and are predicted to do better with hearing aids. The reverse is expected for people who do not accept background noise (Nabelek et al. 2004). Because ANL is a new measure, its predictive value for determining hearing aid satisfaction is not yet known. Considering that background noise is a frequent complaint of hearing aid users, we are likely to hear more about the concept of ANL in the future.

Insurance versus Self-Pay

One of the most interesting findings with regard to satisfaction with hearing aids is that people who have insurance coverage that pays for their hearing aids tend to be more satisfied than are those who must pay all or part of the cost themselves (Cox and Alexander 2001; Faiers and McCarthy 2004). This finding suggests that the greatest way to improve hearing aid satisfaction may not be a matter of technology but a matter of financing.

Concluding Remarks about Hearing Aid Satisfaction

Although the benefits of hearing aids for users can easily be quantified, satisfaction is more abstract and harder to predict. It can sometimes be directly tied to benefits and at other times not. There are technological and user-related factors that have been associated with hearing aid satisfaction, but there is no direct one-to-one relation. Even complete insurance coverage that increases the likelihood of satisfaction with hearing aids does not guarantee satisfaction. The one thing that all the research about hearing aid satisfaction has made clear is that satisfaction is a highly individual perception.

If you have difficulty hearing and are considering the purchase of hearing aids, it is likely they will benefit you; however, the degree to which you will feel satisfied with them is less certain.

7 Non–Hearing Aid Solutions

If a person has a hearing loss that is not medically correctable and does not want to wear hearing aids, there are alternatives for alleviating the listening difficulties and improving his or her ability to communicate. These alternatives are the focus of this chapter.

Common sense changes in behavior can minimize the impact of hearing loss. With a little planning it may be possible to change or avoid difficult listening situations. A variety of technological solutions are also available for specific listening needs. Unfortunately, these possibilities are overlooked. In fact, people frequently act in ways that make it harder for them to hear. Often they do not plan ahead and must endure problematic listening situations because they did not think beforehand about how to cope. These self-defeating habits have been the modus operandi of previous generations. Baby boomers can do better.

The non–hearing aid solutions discussed in this chapter can be of tremendous help to a person with a slight hearing loss that is not bad enough to require hearing aids. They can also be helpful to someone with a mild or more severe loss who could wear hearing aids but does not. Even people who wear hearing aids can benefit from some of these strategies and technologies to maximize their ability to hear. As explained previously, hearing aids do not completely compensate for a hearing loss. The information provided here can help a person to bridge the gap between what hearing aids can do and the listening difficulties that may remain. Conversely, people with normal hearing can use some of this information to avoid self-defeating listening habits.

I have divided the non–hearing aid solutions into two general categories, planning ahead and making use of tools and technology.

Having a Plan

The first step in planning a strategy to cope with hearing loss is to identify the situations that are most problematic. For someone with a slight loss, this might only involve one or two situations. The list is likely to grow, however, with more severe losses. It will also vary depending on listening needs. Someone who is retired and relatively inactive socially does not have the same listening needs as a socially active business person. Given identical hearing losses, the latter will struggle more.

If there are only one or two problematic situations on your list, deciding where to start will not be a concern. If you have many difficult situations, start with the ones that you find most troublesome. The remainder can be dealt with once the most aggravating issues have been addressed. Once you address one trouble spot, it often translates into better hearing under different circumstances. For example, a strategy that helps you to hear in a restaurant is also likely to be helpful at a family gathering because the listening situations are in many ways similar. To do best, however, you should still plan for each situation individually.

Getting Closer

To better hear and understand, move closer to the sound source. Doing so will increase the volume. This is an obvious but overlooked technique. As sound waves move farther from a source, their energy is spread out over a larger area. This means that the amount of sound per area (that is, the amount of sound that can go into your ear) will decrease. A fundamental law of physics known as the inverse square law governs the rate at which this happens. Put in audiometric terms, the inverse square law states that as we double the distance, sound volume decreases by 6 dB. For example, at six feet away from a speaker, the sound is 6 dB less than at three feet. At twenty-four feet, the sound is 18 dB less than at three feet. If we apply this 18-dB change to the audiograms shown in chapter 3, it effectively gives a normal-hearing person a mild hearing loss. A mild loss becomes a moderate loss, and so forth. This discussion is somewhat simplified because it does not take reverberation and a number of other acoustical factors into account, but the general relationship still applies.

The inverse square law shows that sitting on the far side of the living room from a source of sound presents the equivalent of a mild hearing loss or compounds an existing hearing loss. If you sit in the back of a church, theater, or other large space, the sound reduction will be even greater. You can easily negate this effect by sitting closer. Don't feel embarrassed to approach event organizers and explain your difficulty. People can't help you unless they know you have a problem. Be an advocate for yourself.

Directing the Sound toward the Listener or Getting in Front of the Sound

The most direct way for sound to reach a listener is in a straight line. If a speaker stands diagonally to you, you may still hear her, but the sound is reduced because to reach you it may travel to the closest wall and bounce back. On the other hand, a person may go unheard because there is no guarantee that the sound will be reflected in your direction. We have all experienced the listening problems this causes. Even someone with normal hearing may have to strain to hear a person who would have been clearly understandable face-to-face.

People frequently try to talk while walking away from each other. They sit beside rather than across from those they would like to hear. They buy portable or monitor-style televisions with speakers facing the side rather than the viewer. These are only a few examples in which disregarding the direction of sound is counterproductive to hearing. If you look at the situations in which you struggle most, you will likely find that in at least a few of them, you will hear better if you can get in front of the sound or direct it toward you.

Reducing Background Noise

Hearing in a noisy room can be difficult even for a person with normal hearing. One sound may mask another, or sounds may blend together, becoming individually indistinguishable. People with hearing loss struggle more. This remains true even when their worse hearing thresholds are taken into account (Needleman and Crandell 1995). In a background of speech sounds, people with hearing loss have been found to need a signal-to-noise ratio that is 5 to15 dB higher than that needed by normal hearing subjects (Wilson 2003). Finding a way to reduce background noise will improve the signal-to-noise ratio and consequently speech understanding.

For example, at a restaurant, request to be seated in the quieter dining room rather than in the bar. A booth in a corner or against a wall will likely be quieter than a table in the middle of the room surrounded by other diners. A restaurant will be quieter during off hours than during the middle of the lunch or dinner rush. While driving a car, you will more easily hear the radio or passengers if you roll up the windows. In the kitchen, it will be harder to hear while the dishwasher or garbage disposal is on. Just sitting next to a furnace or air conditioning vent can present a problem if the noise from the blower interferes with what you are trying to hear. Recognizing and then minimizing these competing sounds can make a big difference in how well you hear and understand.

A secondary source of unwanted noise can come from reverberation. Sound is reflected off walls and other hard surfaces to be heard as a series of disruptive echoes. Along with background noise, reverberation is another environmental factor that has been shown to negatively impact speech understanding (Cox et al. 1987). The negative effect becomes especially pronounced with advancing age (Harris and Reitz 1985; Divenyi and Haupt 1997). When background noise and reverberation are combined, the unfortunate result for hearing is often referred to as the "cafeteria or cocktail party effect."

Reverberation can be minimized in the home through the use of carpets, curtains, fabrics, and materials that soak up excess sound, such as echoes that can interfere with hearing. Away from the home, reverberation is more problematic because it is harder to control. The cafeteria effect can be so great in some buildings that your best option may be to perform a similar activity in a less reverberant setting. If you need to be in an environment full of echoes, try to do so at a less busy time so that there is less sound to be reflected and cause a listening problem.

Using Lipreading

Most of us use lipreading to some extent. When watching Sunday football on television, you may try to read a coach's lips when the quarterback fumbles the ball, or you may attempt to understand your teenager's mumbled comment after being grounded. Lipreading is typically used to help fill in missing parts when listening to soft or indistinct speech. The human brain does this automatically as part of the speech-understanding process. Just as each consonant or vowel has a distinct sound, there are specific lip movements that are required to produce each. Some overlap in lip movements makes a few speech sounds visually indistinguishable from others, including the letters *p* and *m*. Saying *pan* and *man* in front of a mirror quickly confirms that these consonants look the same when spoken. Although overlaps such as this make lipreading an enhancer and not a substitute for hearing, it remains tremendously helpful for augmenting hearing.

Lipreading can be particularly helpful for understanding in noise. This is true whether speech is indistinct due to background noise or reverberation. Less well recognized is that lipreading cues can also help a person to separate one voice from competing voices (Helfer and Freyman 2005). By focusing on the speech sounds that are temporally related to lip movements, the brain can better focus on one voice within a group. In other words, lipreading may not only help you to better understand but also to better hear.

To lip-read you need to be able to see the person speaking. Having the person close and in good lighting helps. Try not to have the speaker silhouetted by light, as might happen if he or she is seated in front of a window on a bright day. Your lipreading will improve with practice. If you feel the need for a more structured program, you should be able to find a book that teaches lipreading in your local library or bookstore.

Informing Others about Your Hearing Difficulty

Let others help you. Explaining to friends and relatives that you have some hearing loss and that you understand better in certain situations will help them be attentive to your listening needs. You can casually mention that you hear better when sound is coming directly toward you or when there is little background noise, or you might do the reverse and mention that you can't hear when someone is far away or calling from another room. This makes people aware of your hearing problem and how they might help if they are so inclined. Given this knowledge, there is a good chance that many will do what they can to help without directly being asked. Of course this doesn't mean you should hold them responsible for your hearing difficulties. The difference may seem subtle but in reality it is huge.

Using Sign Language

A different way to cope with hearing loss is to forgo spoken language and instead use sign language. This is a very real option as demonstrated by the many people in the deaf community who use sign language as their primary mode of communication. American Sign Language can be learned at universities and community colleges, or with the aid of one of the numerous do-it-yourself books on the subject.

Changing to sign language can be difficult, however, for someone who has communicated his or her whole life through the spoken word. One major misconception about American Sign Language is that it is a simple picture-like language that is easily learned. In actuality, it is a complex language full of nuance and subtlety. Extensive exposure and practice are required for mastery beyond a basic level (Kemp 1998). An individual is unlikely to gain fluency from a single course or from a quick reading of a text.

A bigger issue with regard to sign language may be one of audience. Even if you learn sign language, with whom will you use it? Does your spouse understand sign language? What about your children, friends, co-workers, or customers? What is the chance they will learn? Learning to sign might be like purchasing a telephone calling plan that only lets you connect with people you do not know.

Deciding to use sign language instead of spoken language is a less realistic decision for people who have spent their whole life communicating verbally. Fluency will not be acquired without effort. What's more, it will be easier to make new friends who know how to sign rather than teaching sign language to existing friends. Given some consideration, most people opt for listening strategies, hearing aids, or other assistive technologies that demand fewer lifestyle changes.

Having the Tools

Although getting closer, reducing background noise, and employing other listening strategies are helpful, they are not always adequate without additional tools. Assistive devices for people with hearing loss can be divided into two general categories: devices designed to alert a person to a particular event and tools for improving communication more generally.

Alerting Devices

A person with normal hearing usually takes environmental sounds for granted and doesn't realize his dependence on sounds. Microwave ovens buzz when done. Automatic bread machines beep when it is time to add ingredients. Teakettles whistle. Egg timers ding. These are just a few examples from the kitchen. Hearing loss mutes these and other more important signals such as fire alarms, carbon monoxide detectors, and doorbells.

Doorbell. The standard chiming doorbell is ineffectual for people with hearing loss, especially since the melodic tones are often too soft to hear. Visitors come and go at the door undetected. Fortunately, there are several alternatives to the standard chime doorbell. Perhaps the simplest alternative is to go retro and install a mechanical bell-and-clapper-style ringer. This rather loud "fire station" bell is available at most home improvement centers. Many people who cannot hear a chime doorbell easily hear this distinct ring. Also, some doorbell signalers made for the hearing impaired can be adjusted to ring at different frequencies. A person with a high-frequency hearing loss would set the doorbell to ring at low frequencies, while a person with a low-frequency hearing loss would do the reverse. There are also doorbell signalers that flash a light in place of, or in addition to, an audible sound.

Alarm clock. The alarm clock is another essential household item that is designed for people who hear. Although some individuals have a good internal clock that allows them to wake at the same time everyday, the majority rely on an alarm to ensure they are prompt for appointments, work, and other time-sensitive commitments. People with a mild or moderate hearing loss may need to find a louder alarm clock. Some are naturally loud, such as a wind-up bell-and-clapper-style alarm, while others have an adjustable volume. There are clocks made specifically for the hearing impaired, such as the Sonic Boom alarm clock that is nearly as loud as the name implies. Audible alarms—even very loud ones—can be ineffective for waking someone with a severe or profound hearing loss. For these people, an alarm clock with a pillow vibrator may be the best solution, especially since it spares the ears of a spouse sleeping nearby.

Burglar, fire, carbon monoxide, and other alarms. Every house and apartment should have a fire alarm. Similarly, carbon monoxide detectors are a good idea in buildings with gas heat, fireplaces, or other fossil fuel devices. Many people purchase burglar alarms to feel safe and secure at home, and there are a variety of specialty alarms such as weather radios and baby monitors. All of these alarms are typically auditory.

Purchasing alarms with an extra loud warning is one way people with hearing loss cope with this problem. Switching to a flashing alerting signal is another alternative. Some of these are designed to strobe brightly at a frequency that will awaken a sleeper. Unfortunately, these alarms are still likely to go unheard or unseen from a different part of the house. A single screaming alarm easily alerts a normal hearing person even rooms away, but possibly not someone with hearing loss. To be truly effective, the alerting signal needs to be detectable in every room. This requires the use of a holistic system that sets off the alarm everywhere, even if the area affected may be on the other side of the house. Multiple display panels that indicate what the alarm is and where it originated are also helpful. People with hearing loss frequently place a loud or flashing fire detector in their bedroom and feel this makes them safe, but they overlook the possibility that a fire could start elsewhere in the house and be out of control before their room alarm detects it.

A nontechnological way to be alerted to alarms, signals, and environmental events is to use a trained hearing dog, discussed in box 7.1.

Improving Communication

As mentioned previously, the major quality-of-life detriments caused by a hearing loss result from communication difficulties. Hearing

Box 7.1. Hearing dogs

The use of guide dogs is well recognized as a way to improve mobility and safety for the visually impaired or blind. Less recognized is the use of specially trained dogs to help the hearing impaired. These "hearing dogs" assist the deaf and hard of hearing by alerting them to a variety of sounds. A few of these sounds might include the ringing of a doorbell or a knock at the door, the ringing of a telephone, or the sounding of a smoke or fire alarm. Hearing dogs can even be trained to alert a hearing-impaired person to the sound of a baby crying. In response to one of these sounds, the dog makes physical contact and leads the individual to the sound source. Hearing dogs can help a person with hearing loss to maintain independence and to feel more confident and secure. A number of organizations train hearing dogs. If you are interested in this service, talk with a hearing professional in your area.

loss can leave a person feeling isolated. Improving the ability to communicate in just a few situations such as during telephone conversations, at public concerts or lectures, and while watching television can help reduce feelings of isolation and other negative consequences of a hearing loss.

Telephone. The telephone presents one of the more difficult listening challenges for a person with hearing loss. Although the sound is usually very clear (some cordless and cellular phones excluded), the volume is not always loud enough for someone with hearing difficulties to hear the softest consonant sounds. The problem is worse because of the use of only one ear and the lack of lipreading cues that could augment hearing in face-to-face conversations. Fortunately, there are several options to improve hearing and understanding on the phone.

Replacing an existing phone with the old corded styles such as those used by AT&T or Bell Telephone may be the first step to a better phone experience in that some of the inexpensive contemporary models provide a poorer reproduction of sound. Sound reproduction on a cordless phone can also be worse, depending on the quality of the phone and the amount of local radio interference. The quality of sound on a cellular phone can vary between analog and digital phones and by the local signal strength. In general, cell phones and cordless models make it harder to hear, and a person with hearing loss cannot afford to start with sound that is less than perfect. You need to be selective in the phones you use. If you cannot hear on any standard phone (corded, cordless, or cellular), then you may need one made specifically for people with hearing loss.

Many electronics stores sell telephones made specifically for the hearing impaired: the volume is adjustable, and on some models the frequency response can be altered. These phones are also available from various audiology and hearing aid centers, but the price is often higher than in retail stores.

Using a headset made for the telephone is another option. These are common in business, where a telephone receptionist or customer service specialist needs to be able to talk on the phone and have his or her hands free to type or write. The model used in business typically covers one ear and has a small microphone in front to speak into. The listening volume is adjustable. For someone with hearing loss, a headset that covers both ears literally doubles the chance to hear and is widely available for purchase.

In fact, my patient Patty, who was mentioned in chapter 1, benefited from an amplified telephone headset that covered one ear. As you may recall, she was having trouble at her job in an auto parts shop due to her hearing difficulty. The amplified headset allowed her to better hear phone orders for auto parts and left her hands free to record sales. She then wore a hearing aid in the opposite ear to hear co-workers and walk-in customers.

There are also alternatives to standard telephone conversations, for example, a telephone device for the deaf (TDD). A TDD is also known as a text telephone or more commonly as a teletypewriter (TTY), a special kind of typewriter that connects directly to the phone line. A person communicates by typing on a TTY, which sends the text message in real time to another person with a TTY. The message is displayed on the receiver's TTY, who can then respond in kind. Many businesses have a separate phone number for TTY users.

Friends and family members of a hearing-impaired person with a TTY sometimes purchase one for themselves to make two-way communication possible.

It might at first seem that a TTY would be of limited use if only one party has this technology. A TTY cannot communicate with a regular phone. Fortunately, there are relay services that you can call with a TTY that will then talk over the phone with the person you wish to contact. The relay service acts as an intermediary in the conversation. Someone who wishes to talk with you can also call the relay service, which will then communicate with you through your TTY. The phone book should have a listing for relay services as well as for local businesses that have a TTY phone number.

Text messaging is another alternative for communicating through the phone. Today's cellular phones have a small display screen on which short text messages can be viewed. Messages can be written by entering letters on the phone keypad. You would not want to carry on a lengthy discussion in this manner but it can work well for short messages. Text messaging has become a fad for teenagers, but it can be a practical asset for the hearing impaired. Another useful feature of cell phones is the vibrating ringer. These two features combined reduce the risk that a call will be missed or misunderstood.

Finally, computer e-mail and instant messaging offer other alternatives to the telephone. The information exchanged in many phone conversations could just as easily be carried out through e-mail. Unlike TTYs, personal computers are widespread so there is less concern about an intended recipient lacking the necessary technology. E-mail interactions may be less spontaneous than phone conversations, but they are unambiguous. If a discussion needs to be carried out in real time, it can be conducted on a computer by using instant messaging or some other form of computer chat.

Understanding messages left on a phone answering machine can be another challenge. Although answering machines can sometimes be turned up loud enough for a person with hearing loss, the sound quality usually suffers. Fortunately there are amplified phone machines that are designed to play more loudly. On a few models it is even possible to slow down the playback of the recording to try to make fast speech more distinct.

Television. Some of the same listening strategies that make it easier to hear during one-on-one conversations are often helpful while watching television. Getting closer, watching the person speaking, and reducing background noise are particularly key. You may also want to consider investing in a larger television, since lipreading is more easily accomplished on a larger screen and reading closed-captioning is also easier.

Perhaps the simplest way to optimize television sound is to use headphones. This puts the sound directly into your ears without background noise. It also eliminates any problems caused by poor room acoustics. If you are fortunate enough to have a tone control or separate bass and treble controls on your television, adjust the television for the sound balance that is most understandable. Since high-frequency hearing loss is most common, it is likely you will do best by emphasizing the treble and minimizing the bass sounds. If you have worse hearing at the low frequencies, the reverse may be true.

One of the great misconceptions involving television is that stereo sound or surround sound will always be more understandable than a monaural signal. This is unfortunately not true since television manufacturers often add a bass boost to the stereo or surround-sound settings to create a deeper, more pleasing sound that is harder for many people with hearing problems to understand. Furthermore, too many low-frequency sounds may mask high-frequency sounds, thereby interfering with word understanding. Sound from the multiple speakers in surround-sound systems can also interact with room acoustics, creating reverberation. You may find that for understandability, adjusting your television sound settings to monaural listening may work best.

Personal devices for multiple listening situations. A device that helps with the television or telephone can be a tremendous help, but only for those specific uses. There are, however, devices that can help in multiple situations, such as a personal amplifier. A personal amplifier looks similar to a Walkman radio and would likely be indistinguishable from one to a casual observer. Miniature headphones or ear buds are connected by a wire to the main part of the device, which is clipped to a belt or worn in a pocket. The unit has an adjustable volume control and, on some models, a tone control. If there are times when you would like to be able to turn people louder, like you do the television set, a personal amplifier gives you this option. Although most of these devices tend to amplify speech and noise alike, they can still be helpful. Basic models are relatively inexpensive and can usually be purchased from a local electronics store.

A personal FM system—a device that consists of a small FM radio transmitter and receiver—employs a different strategy to help with hearing impairment. The transmitter is placed on or near the sound source, and the listener wears the receiver. The goal is to amplify specific sounds and is the technological equivalent of getting as close as possible to the person speaking. Because the transmitter is small, someone else can wear it. This could allow you to hear your spouse if he or she is across the room, talking in a different direction, or calling from the other end of the house. FM systems are available for both general and specific listening needs. Many systems are also compatible with hearing aids. An audiologist would be able to help select a system that would work best for your listening needs.

Amplified earmuffs are another personal device that can have a listening benefit in a variety of settings. This special form of hearing protection adjusts loud sounds to a safe level while allowing the wearer to adjust softer sounds to an audible volume. Traditional earplugs tend to block everything: they reduce loud sounds to a safe level but then leave normal conversational speech inaudible. A hunter may want to hear the sounds of approaching game yet still have protection against the crack of a rifle or shotgun. A woodworker may want to hear the radio between saw cuts or hammer blows without constantly having to remove earplugs. There are a number of situations such as these in which electronic earmuffs not only provide hearing protection but also an improved chance to hear. This relatively new form of protective hearing device is available at gun shops and some home improvement centers.

Improved listening in public places. In 1990, the U.S. Congress passed the Americans with Disabilities Act (ADA) with the intent that businesses, schools, government, and public venues should make reasonable accommodations for people with disabilities, including people with hearing loss. The manner in which the law is implemented can vary greatly, depending on the specific situation. With regard to hearing, compliance might range from giving preferential seating to a person with hearing loss to providing a sign language interpreter for those who communicate in this manner. More often, some form of assistive listening device is employed. It could be as basic as loaning a personal amplifier to a customer or guest. In a lecture hall or theater, a number of seats may be wired for amplified headphones. FM and other wireless listening systems are also frequently employed. Some of these options can be used alone or along with hearing aids.

In effect, you need not own an assistive listening device to benefit from one. However, you must be willing to ask if assistive listening accommodations are available. This help is often on hand but rarely advertised. There will be no flashing neon sign saying "Assistive Listening Devices Here."

8 New and Future Options

Baby boomers have options for coping with a hearing loss that were not available to their parents or grandparents. This chapter presents new, significantly improved, and promising medical and technological options for coping with hearing loss. Some of these alternatives will sound familiar; others will not. These new choices are grouped into the categories of prevention, surgery, hearing aids, and a possible cure.

Current treatments are often the result of small improvements in existing therapies. A surgery that has been performed for many years may be more successful today than in the past, even though it is essentially the same surgery. What makes this possible is some small incremental change in procedure or technique.

Stapedectomy, for example, was described in chapter 4 as a highly successful surgical treatment for conductive hearing losses resulting from otosclerosis. In a small percentage of patients, however, the initial surgery is unsuccessful. When this occurs, hearing can often be restored through a second surgery. One study showed that the use of a new surgical device known as the argon laser improved the overall success rate of second surgeries by 10 percent. In select cases in which the laser was especially helpful, the success rate jumped more than 20 percent (Lippy et al. 2003). Similar advances in other areas of hearing healthcare have occurred and are making just as much difference.

Prevention

Obviously prevention is the best option, especially considering that there is no cure for sensorineural hearing loss. New technologies and advances in medicine make it easier to detect signs of initial loss and then prevent them before they become serious problems.

Otoacoustic Emissions

One of the detection methods is based on the knowledge that the healthy ear "talks back" to incoming sounds and also makes noise on its own. In the late 1970s David Kemp (1978, 1979) reported that he was able to detect very soft sounds coming from the inner ear of normal hearing subjects. Some of these sound emissions occurred in response to outside sound, whereas others occurred spontaneously. It seemed that if you sang to an ear, it would sing back. If you did not sing, the ear might still sing to itself. The traditional view of ear mechanics held that the inner ear was passive and only acted to process sound. It should not sing. The concept of the inner ear as a passive system was debunked for good when research showed that outer hair cells could move on their own (Brownell 1984; Brownell et al. 1985).

In the mid- to late 1990s, what was by then known as otoacoustic emissions (OAEs) had become the hottest thing in hearing science. During this decade OAEs were investigated or used in more than a thousand scientific studies. The outer-hair-cell movement that Brownell observed in the 1980s became accepted as the source of OAEs. Clinical OAE test equipment was developed and found its way to research facilities, hospitals, and audiology and otology practices. Knowledge about OAEs grew quickly, and the presence or absence of these emissions from an ear became widely recognized as having diagnostic value.

One of the first and most widespread uses of OAE testing was to determine hearing loss in infants and very young children. In the absence of ear infections or other peripheral pathology, children with normal hearing almost always have measurable OAEs. Children with a slight or mild hearing loss can also have measurable OAEs, but the response is usually not as robust. No OAEs are expected for more severe hearing losses. OAE testing has become the standard of care for screening the hearing of infants in hospital nurseries.

For baby boomers, the greatest value of OAE testing lies in monitoring the ear for damaging effects from noise or harmful substances.

OAE testing is so sensitive that it can detect inner ear damage not found through conventional audiometry (Attias et al. 2001; Lucertini et al. 2002). Although some researchers are still recommending further study of OAEs to determine what role the emissions may play in hearing conservation programs (Lapsley Miller et al. 2004; Seixas et al. 2004), the evidence is mounting that the role will be huge.

The test itself is quick and painless. It involves sitting quietly for several minutes while an audiologist places a noisy earplug in an ear. The ear listens to the test equipment, and the test equipment in turn listens to the ear. The results are printed out and interpreted immediately. They can also be saved and compared over time. OAE testing is of little or no benefit if a person already has a significant hearing loss because the ear will no longer produce otoacoustic emissions. If a person has normal or near-normal hearing, however, OAE testing may make it possible to recognize and act on the first signs of nerve damage from noise or chemical exposure before the person's hearing is affected.

Medicines to Prevent Noise-Induced Hearing Loss

Preliminary research suggests that medicine might one day be an alternative to earplugs or earmuffs to protect against loud noise. A number of substances investigated through animal research have been reported to provide at least some protection from noise trauma. A few of these promising substances include magnesium (Scheibe et al. 2001), ebselen (Pourbakht and Yamasoba 2003), caroverine (Chen et al. 2004), and N-L-acetylcysteine (Duan et al. 2004). Chemical combinations have also been examined and reported to provide significant protection from continuous and short-impulsive noise (Hight et al. 2003).

Magnesium is one of the few substances reported to have a protective effect in humans. In placebo-controlled double-blind studies, magnesium was found to offer protection against the temporary (Attias et al. 2004) and permanent (Attias et al. 1994) hearing losses that can result from excessive noise. Although it is still too early to give up earplugs or earmuffs for a pharmaceutical alternative, this could eventually become a possibility for many baby boomers.

Surgery

In addition to the argon laser mentioned earlier, there are many other small procedural and prosthetic innovations that have made a difference in improving hearing. What's more, advancements in medical imaging have reduced the need for exploratory surgeries and the risk of unexpected complications. A few recent innovations involve a combination of surgery and technology. One advance restores hearing to the deaf. The other improves hearing for a group of people who were told for years that nothing could help their inability to hear.

Cochlear Implants

A cochlear implant is an electronic device that restores hearing to people with severe or profound sensorineural hearing loss. It consists of two parts, an internal device (fig. 8.1) that is surgically implanted behind the ear between the skin and mastoid bone and an externally worn sound processor (fig. 8.2). A small electrode array extends from the body of the internal device into the curved space of the inner ear. Some models also have a separate ball or reference electrode that is placed under one of the jaw muscles. The internal device is designed to last a lifetime.

The external device is worn over the ear, much like a behind-the-ear hearing aid. Batteries that power the implant are housed in the external sound processor and can easily be changed by the wearer. If after years of use the external device wears out and needs to be

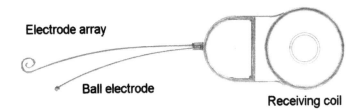

Figure 8.1. Surgically implanted portion of a cochlear implant.

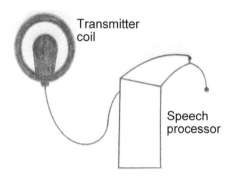

Figure 8.2. Externally worn cochlear implant sound processor.

replaced, a new updated sound processor can be purchased to work with the existing internal device.

A cochlear implant does not work by making sound louder. Instead, a cochlear implant works by electrically stimulating the nerves underlying the damaged inner ear hair cells and becomes a substitute for them. A small microphone on the sound processor collects sound, which the external sound processor codes. This coded signal is sent to a coil held in place by a magnet directly over the internal device. Sound is transmitted from the coil to the internal device through magnetic induction. The internal device then distributes this signal to the individual electrodes within the electrode array. Exactly how sound is coded and distributed among electrodes varies between implant manufacturers. It also varies from person to person, depending on the extent of nerve damage among other factors. Consequently, cochlear implants need to be individually programmed for each recipient.

Early cochlear implants were considered a success if they could provide the awareness of sound and some help with lipreading. Understanding without lipreading was not the expectation. Even so, the restoration of any amount of hearing was a miracle for those who had been previously deaf. Over time and through technological advances, the implants have become more effective. The expectation today is that the wearer is able to understand conversations without the help of lipreading. Sentence recognition without lipreading has advanced to an average of about 86 percent for those who have some newer implant models (Higgins et al. 2002; Pasanisi et al. 2003). When profoundly deaf persons who use hearing aids are compared with those who use a cochlear implant, the hearing performance of implant users is clearly superior when they are listening in both quiet and noisy environments (Hamzavi et al. 2001).

Cochlear implants provide an improved quality of life. One study showed that 96 percent of implant patients studied reported an overall quality-of-life improvement (Higgins et al. 2002). A separate study found that the greatest quality-of-life benefits were related to improved communication, reduction in feelings of being a burden, less isolation, and improved relations with family and friends (Mo et al. 2005). Family and friends also reported an improved quality of life as a result of their loved one's implant.

One recent advance in cochlear implant systems is that the implant itself can be used to assess the responsiveness of the inner ear to electrical stimulation. This process is called neural response telemetry (NRT) and offers great promise for programming the implant as well as for providing information about the status of the internal device and auditory nerves (Di Nardo et al. 2003; Kiss et al. 2003; Charasse et al. 2004). Cochlear implants have traditionally been programmed for each user on something of a trial-and-error basis. Each electrode is turned on individually, and the patient describes when the sound produced is audible, comfortable, or uncomfortably loud. This process usually produces a hearing result that is optimized for an individual. Although this may not seem like a difficult task to someone with normal hearing, it can be difficult for a person who has been living without sound. When there is doubt about how an implant should be adjusted, NRT can provide an objective basis for programming. It seems likely that using the information provided by NRT along with patient responses may ultimately result in an even better hearing outcome.

Bone-Anchored Hearing Aid System

A different fusion of surgery and technology is employed with a bone-anchored hearing aid (BAHA). Candidates for the BAHA include persons with a conductive hearing loss whose problem cannot otherwise be surgically corrected and persons with single-sided

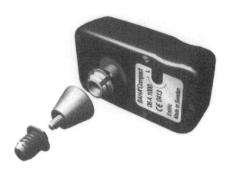

Figure 8.3. Parts of the BAHA system. Courtesy of Entific Medical Systems

sensorineural deafness. Many BAHA candidates with conductive hearing loss may have already undergone several unsuccessful ear surgeries and been told that further procedures would not be helpful. Until very recently, candidates with single-sided deafness were told that there was no help beyond the CROS hearing aid described in chapter 5. The BAHA system provides the prospect of improved hearing for each of these groups.

The BAHA system consists of three parts (fig. 8.3). The first is a small threaded titanium implant that is surgically placed into the bone behind the ear. A cone-shaped titanium abutment is connected to the implant and protrudes slightly from the skin. Connected to the abutment is a detachable sound processor. The titanium implant is placed into the skull during an outpatient procedure that is typically performed under local anesthesia. The abutment is connected to the implant during the surgery but may be connected later in special cases. A period of two to three months is allowed for the surrounding bone to fuse with the implant through a process known as osseointegration. The sound processor can be attached after this period.

The BAHA works through bone-conducted sound. The process involved is similar to the pure-tone bone conduction audiometry test that was described in chapter 3. Sound vibrations are sent directly through the skull to the inner ear. The BAHA is more efficient, however, because the processor is coupled directly to the skull. There is no intervening skin to attenuate sound. Figure 8.4 shows how the BAHA would work for someone who is deaf in the left ear. The pro-

Left   **Right**

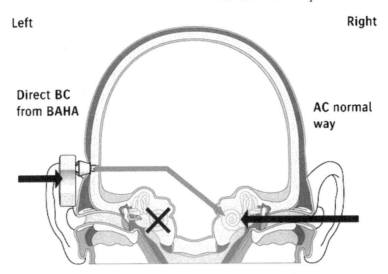

Direct BC
from BAHA

AC normal
way

Figure 8.4. BAHA sound transmission for single-sided deafness. Courtesy of Entific Medical Systems

cessor is worn on the nonhearing left side and transmits sound directly through the skull to the normal-hearing right ear. Although sound from the BAHA would reach the left inner ear, this nonfunctional ear does not process the sound. It is the right ear that is doing the work. Although the BAHA uses the good ear, it does not interfere with it. Sound coming from the right still enters the ear normally.

For someone with a conductive hearing loss, the BAHA bypasses any peripheral malformation or damage, and sound is heard on the same side as the processor. The BAHA can restore normal hearing sensitivity to people who have up to a severe conductive hearing loss.

Unambiguous benefits with the BAHA have been reported for conductive and single-sided hearing losses. Hearing handicap is significantly reduced in each of these cases (Wazen et al. 2001). Reported satisfaction with the BAHA is high for persons with conductive hearing loss (Lustig et al. 2001) and for those with single-sided deafness (Wazen et al. 2003). When compared with the other alternative for single-sided deafness (a CROS hearing aid), greater benefit has been reported with the BAHA (Wazen et al. 2003).

Hearing Aids

Hearing aid manufacturers constantly advertise that they have developed some new innovation that is the latest and greatest. It can be difficult to differentiate between hyped advertisement and actual advancement. I have highlighted a few of the more recent and ongoing innovations that are worthy of notice.

Directional Microphones

A directional microphone improves hearing by allowing the person to focus on sound from one area rather than having to hear above competing sounds. Traditionally, a directional microphone is oriented in a hearing aid so that it detects sound in front of the listener. Although this process worked well in the laboratory, results were mixed in outside conditions. Real people have the annoying habit of not always being in front of the listener or of walking as they talk, resulting in speakers being outside the range of the directional microphone and going unheard.

A smarter technology that automatically searches and focuses on people speaking makes the directional microphone more effective. In 2004, researchers reported that a three-microphone hearing aid system "allowed a group of hearing-impaired individuals with mild-to-moderate sensorineural hearing loss to perform similarly to young, normal-hearing individuals" (Bentler et al. 2004). Smart directional microphones such as this are likely to become an integral part of future hearing aid designs. My colleagues and I recommended this option for Kathie, who was the funeral home operator mentioned in chapter 1. This gave her the chance to understand better at work and in her social life.

Digital Feedback Suppression

An occasional but annoying side effect of a hearing aid is the loud whistling sound created when sound exiting the hearing aid does not stay in the ear but finds its way into the hearing aid microphone to start a feedback cycle. It is a common problem when a hearing aid fits the ear poorly, is turned on too loud, or is covered by an obstruction such as a hand, hat, or scarf. Reducing the hearing aid volume reduces or eliminates feedback at the expense of hearing. Making a hearing aid fit the ear more snuggly could better keep sound from escaping, but this is at the expense of comfort.

By the 1990s research showed that it was possible to build an active feedback suppression system into digital hearing aids. The technology reduced the likelihood of feedback with little or no corresponding reduction in performance. In fact, aided hearing ability was likely to improve because the hearing aids could be turned louder when needed. Digital feedback suppression (DFS) makes possible an additional 10 to 18 dB of sound before feedback becomes problematic (Dyrlund and Bisgaard 1991; Joson et al. 1993; Dyrlund et al. 1994). Although a number of technical details make it nearly impossible to completely eliminate the chance of feedback, DFS greatly reduces it.

DFS is also helpful with the telephone. Because a telephone handset bounces sound back toward a hearing aid, anyone without a telecoil has an increased risk of feedback. Not only does DFS reduce the annoyance of feedback when using the phone, but it also results in improved speech understanding because the aid does not need to be turned down when using the phone (Latzel et al. 2001).

Some form of DFS is now included on most high-end digital hearing aids. The technology is beginning to filter down into mid- and entry-level digitals, and this feature will likely become the rule rather than the exception.

Open Ear Acoustics

The physical presence of hearing aids in the ears can change the subjective sound of a person's own voice and is a common complaint for hearing aid users. The sensation is called the occlusion effect and is typically likened to the sound of talking in a barrel. You can easily experience this sensation by sticking a finger in each ear and speaking aloud. Notice how the sound seems to reverberate in your head. Is it any wonder that a hearing aid wearer might complain?

The best way to prevent the occlusion effect is to leave the ear canal as open as possible. Including a large vent that extends through the length of the hearing aid is one way to achieve this end. Using some form of open non-occluding earmold is another. Unfortunately, this increases the likelihood that sound will escape the ear to produce feedback. Until recently there was no good way to overcome this drawback. The development of DFS changed this. It is now often possible to cancel out feedback as soon as it starts. The result has been a variety of new hearing aid and earmold models that do not block the ear. Consequently, the wearer can have improved hearing without this negative side effect.

Smarter Hearing Aids

Digital hearing aids are little computers. Their overall sophistication and processing power continue to improve. In fact some manufacturers are beginning to advertise their high-end products as having artificial intelligence. Although this may sound far-fetched, digital hearing aids "decide" how to optimize an individual's hearing. The digital aid can adjust and account for hearing loss, loudness sensitivity, listening preferences, and a moment-by-moment analysis of the wearer's listening environment. The greater the hearing aid memory and processing speed, the more variables that can be taken into account.

Future hearing aids may be designed to learn from the user. A hearing aid wearer might use a program button to manually select the memory setting or microphone type that seems optimal in a variety of environments. If later confronted with similar circumstances, the hearing aid would automatically make the required adjustment. Some high-tech hearing aids currently track the amount of time the wearer uses each program in order to help hearing professionals with programming decisions.

Speech Recognition Software

The use of a computer and speech recognition software is yet another way to enhance a person's hearing. This software can be used to automatically convert spoken language into text. Although the know-how to do this has been around for years, it was not until recently that home computers gained the processing speed to quickly perform this conversion. Incoming speech has to be digitized and compared with an extensive record of stored speech sounds. Depending on the computer speed, this process can take time. Most new computers can make the speech-to-text conversion in real time.

Another snag that has slowed the development of speech recognition software has been accuracy. The software can misinterpret what is said because of variations in pronunciation and dialect as well as words that may sound the same but are spelled differently. Advances have also been made in this area, but 100 percent accuracy remains elusive.

The primary application for speech recognition software has been as a replacement for typing. It has also been proposed as a solution for nontypists and as a business alternative to using a transcriptionist. There are now several commercial and home speech recognition packages available for these purposes. To my knowledge, there is not currently a speech recognition system designed specifically for the hearing impaired. In the future, however, there almost certainly will be. The potential benefits are clear for talking on the phone and listening to voice mail or a phone-answering machine. In one-on-one conversations the device might effectively provide the listener with subtitles. Those who are not afraid to experiment may be able to adapt one of the current systems for their own. The rest of us will likely have to wait for one of the software giants to accomplish this.

Speech recognition software may one day be the magic bullet for the hearing impaired, just as word processing and spreadsheet programs greatly enhanced the abilities of business professionals.

A Cure

The real goal with regard to hearing loss is to find a cure. Prevention is a nice idea, but it doesn't correct an existing loss. Hearing aids may help, but they are certainly no cure. Most ear surgeries are performed to remedy a conductive hearing loss—not the sensorineural losses that are responsible for the vast majority of hearing problems. Ear surgeries such as cochlear implants that are performed for sensorineural loss are not so much a cure as a way to bypass existing damage. The bottom line with hearing loss is that most losses are the result of nerve damage that is currently viewed as irreversible. With the advent of new technologies, this view may soon change.

Nerve Cell Regeneration

It is correctly believed that nerve cell development in the inner ear ends shortly before birth. Nerves that are damaged after this time do not recover, making hearing loss permanent. In 1987, two unrelated scientific studies contradicted this belief by presenting evidence that nerve cell regeneration in the inner ear is possible.

The first study examined the course of nerve damage caused by the ototoxic medication gentamicin (Cruz et al. 1987). Healthy chicks were given a course of the drug and then sacrificed so that the inner ear could be microscopically examined. Chicks that were examined right after treatment showed the greatest inner ear damage. Those that were sacrificed and examined two weeks later exhibited partial hair cell restoration.

Another study looked at the effect of noise trauma on the inner ears of chicks. Signs of nerve cell recovery were seen under scanning electron microscopy as early as two days after this trauma. The progression of changes appeared to follow a pattern similar to normal embryologic development (Cotanche 1987).

Findings from these two landmark studies were quickly replicated in chicks and other birds (Corwin and Cotanche 1988; Ryals and Rubel 1988; Girod et al. 1989). Nerve cell recovery was possible and did in fact occur in the avian inner ear. What's more, the regeneration of nerve cells resulted in dramatic improvements in hearing. Given sufficient time, hearing was either partially (Marean et al. 1993) or almost completely recovered (Tucci and Rubel 1990).

Although the hair cells of mammals, unlike those of birds, do not regenerate spontaneously, there is hope that the cells can be regenerated through scientific intervention, including stem cell grafts and gene therapy. Preliminary research with mice has shown that neural stem cells can successfully be grafted into a mammalian inner ear. It further appears that these transplanted cells are capable of differentiating into nerve cells (Tateya et al. 2003; Hu et al. 2005).

The second method that may prove useful is gene therapy. If the correct gene that regulates cell development and replacement is found, it may be possible to tell healthy nonsensory support cells to change into sensory nerve cells. Recent research with guinea pigs using a gene known as *Math1*, and with rats using the gene *Hath1*, has indicated that the cells in the mammalian inner ear are capable of this transformation (Kawamoto et al. 2003; Shou et al. 2003). Hearing improvements have actually been reported in animals following *Math1* therapy (Izumikawa et al. 2005).

Nerve cell regeneration is in its infancy as a science. It holds great promise, but there are many obstacles yet to overcome. We are not likely to see the advent of human nerve cell regeneration in the short term. The procedure has the potential, however, to become the standard for future hearing care. With continued research, this could possibly occur within the lifetime of many baby boomers.

Getting More Information

Before the Internet, little information about ear disease and hearing loss was readily available to the average person. Pamphlets were available from hearing aid manufacturers, but these were less educational and more focused on marketing. Local libraries might have had limited information on the subject, but their holdings were unlikely to be comprehensive. Bookstores rarely stocked books about hearing loss, so people were often unaware of the existence of texts that might be helpful. Scientific studies were performed, but the results were published in subscription journals that were not accessible to the public. Physicians would diagnose, and when possible, treat hearing loss, but rarely did they have the time to thoroughly address the issue of prevention.

The Internet gives us direct access to a wealth of information relevant to our hearing health. Almost all of the major medical, audiological, and hearing aid organizations have websites that list their services and provide educational materials. Information about hearing-related products is also online. We can easily find out what books are in print on a hearing-related subject by a quick search at one of the online bookstores. Abstracts (summaries) of current research are available through Medline (www.ncbi.nlm.nih.gov/entrez), which is a searchable database of medical studies. If you are concerned that something in your diet, work environment, or lifestyle may put you at risk of hearing loss, searching Medline will alert you to any known associations between the activity or substance and hearing ability. Even your standard Internet browser is an indispensable tool. Type in "hearing loss" and "medicine," "hearing loss" and "noise exposure," or "hearing loss" and "solvents" and see what you find.

A variety of resources for recognizing, preventing, treating, and coping with a hearing loss are listed at the end of the book.

9　The Issues
　　That Remain

The ways in which hearing loss can affect each of us and why we as baby boomers should be concerned are by now apparent. The greatest threats to hearing have been discussed, as well as what can be done to prevent, correct, and compensate for a hearing loss. We have even peered ahead to consider treatments and technology that may be available in the near or distant future. Now, just a few issues remain.

First, there are a few details to consider involving the purchase of the aids. Health insurance as it applies to hearing care and hearing aids is another important concern. Discussions of hearing care thus far have focused on what can be done, but not how to pay for it. Unfortunately, it is the issue of payment that is often the biggest obstacle.

Hearing research is another relevant issue for baby boomers. Earlier generations had a limited interest in hearing research, tending to disregard hearing loss until it was so severe as to no longer be denied. By then, research seemed futile because it could not produce an immediate cure and there was no longer time to wait. In contrast, most baby boomers have time, so there is the possibility of finding a cure before boomers develop a problem.

Finally, I reiterate the importance of taking an active role in your hearing health. This includes the consideration of all options, from prevention and planning to treatment and a possible cure. You can take charge rather than be the victim of circumstance.

Hearing Aids Revisited

The hearing aid purchasing process was briefly described in chapter 5. An audiologist or hearing instrument specialist makes a mold of a person's ear, which is then sent to a hearing aid manufacturer. The manufacturer builds a hearing aid to the exact shape of the ear and incorporates the circuitry and features that have been specified. Programming of the aid is done by the hearing instrument specialist or audiologist. This professional also checks to ensure that the finished product fits the intended ear. Several follow-up visits are customary to fine-tune the initial hearing aid settings based on real-life use. If the hearing aid is unsatisfactory, it can be returned for a refund (minus a trial fee) within a set period of time. If the aid is returned, it is still possible to try a different brand, style, or circuit that may perform better.

Although this lengthy process may produce the optimal hearing result, it is labor intensive and expensive for both the fitter and manufacturer. Not surprisingly, the cost is passed on to the consumer. Unfortunately, the process required does not lend itself to price reductions through economies of scale.

Further complicating the hearing aid buying process is the requirement for a medical evaluation. In 1977 the U.S. Food and Drug Administration (FDA) began requiring a medical evaluation by a physician (preferably an ear specialist) before the purchase of hearing aids. Officials feared that someone with a correctable hearing loss might be sold hearing aids and not informed of the medical alternatives. The medical evaluation also ensures that hearing aids will not be sold to a person who might not need or be able to benefit from them. Still other concerns that led to the requirement of a medical evaluation were that an infection might go untreated, that obvious signs of disease might be missed, or that more serious conditions such as an acoustic tumor might go undiagnosed. Adults with religious, philosophical, or other objections to a medical evaluation were to be given the option of signing a waiver (box 9.1). Hearing aid fitters were tasked with the responsibility of informing people that signing this waiver was not in their best interest. Furthermore, they were specifically prohibited from encouraging people to forgo an evaluation. The waiver was not to be an option for adults who had ear pain, drainage, or other "red flag" symptoms. It was also not an option for children.

The cost and inconvenience of the medical examination and fitting process are a clear disincentive to the purchase of hearing aids.

Box 9.1. Waiver of medical evaluation requirements for a hearing aid (U.S. Food and Drug Administration 1977).

I have been advised by _____ (hearing aid dispenser's name) that the Food and Drug Administration has determined that my best health interest would be served if I had a medical evaluation by a licensed physician (preferably a physician who specializes in diseases of the ear) before purchasing a hearing aid. I do not wish a medical evaluation before purchasing a hearing aid.

A routine medical examination and hearing evaluation at an ear, nose, and throat clinic can cost $200 or more. The price of a hearing aid is in addition to this expense. These costs have led many to ask if there might be some safe yet easier and more efficient way. Two frequent suggestions for solving this problem have been to eliminate the requirement of a medical evaluation and to develop a one-size-fits-all hearing aid that can be purchased over the counter. In fact, the FDA recently reviewed specific proposals addressing each idea.

Hearing Aids and the Requirement of a Medical Examination

On August 8, 2003, audiologist Gail Gudmundsen submitted a citizen petition to the FDA requesting revocation of the medical examination requirement for hearing aids. She asked that the existing language in the code of federal regulations be changed to omit wording stating that it is in a prospective hearing aid user's best interest to first have a medical evaluation. She also proposed that the medical waiver was unnecessary and should be eliminated. In place of these requirements Dr. Gudmundsen proposed giving prospective hearing aid users written information about hearing aids and possible medical concerns or contraindications. The statement would explain that hearing aids do not restore normal hearing or prevent further loss. It would also list specific conditions or symptoms that indicate the need for a medical evaluation.

In the petition, Dr. Gudmundsen argued that to deny people access to hearing aids without a medical evaluation is like denying them the option to buy over-the-counter reading glasses. She further argued that what separates prescription from nonprescription medications is often the potential to do harm if misused. The potential for harm from the direct purchase of a hearing aid, she claimed, was minimal. On the practical side, she insisted that since the vast majority of hearing losses are sensorineural and not medically correctable, having this medical requirement mandates unnecessary medical care.

This was not how the FDA viewed the medical requirement. A summary of the FDA report that denied the petition explained that consumer protection was the underlying concern (Boswell 2004). The medical concerns that led to the 1977 hearing aid rule had not changed. Furthermore, providing a list of "red flag" conditions to a hearing aid purchaser was considered insufficient protection. A person could easily be unaware of any one of these problems, and without medical or audiometric evaluation it would go undiagnosed. Medical assessment was thus affirmed as an important and necessary part of the hearing aid purchasing process.

Although the basic requirement for medical clearance before hearing aid use was set in place with the best intentions, the implementation of this process often fails to meet the intended purpose. The biggest problem is the option of a medical waiver. On the one hand the FDA is saying that a medical examination is vital and required, while on the other hand it is saying that an exam is not needed if a person does not want to have one. The option of a medical waiver also presents hearing aid fitters with a tremendous conflict of interest. This piece of paper may be all that stands between them and a hearing aid sale, yet they are not allowed to encourage a potential hearing aid buyer to sign it.

Eliminating the waiver entirely and requiring everyone to have a medical examination by an otologist or ENT physician before the purchase of hearing aids would be the optimal solution from a medical perspective. It has the potential, however, to further increase cost and lengthen the purchasing process. It is also impractical because the coming influx of hearing-impaired baby boomers will likely overwhelm the limited number of these professionals. One alternative might be found by looking at past practices. In 1977, when the hearing aid rule was enacted, hearing instrument specialists—then known as hearing aid dealers or dispensers—were the primary source for hearing aids. They were not required to have the medical or audiological training that might have helped them to recognize treatable or potentially serious medical conditions related to hearing loss. Consequently, this led to missed diagnoses, delayed diagnoses, and the hearing aid rule.

Audiologists did not begin dispensing hearing aids in large numbers until after 1978. Before this time, the American Speech-Language-Hearing Association (ASHA) forbade audiologists from making a profit on the sale of hearing aids. Not surprisingly, audiologists sold few hearing aids while this edict was in place. A U.S. Supreme Court decision involving the National Society of Engineers (*United States v. National Society of Professional Engineers* 1978) changed all of this when the Court ruled that a society could not limit competition among its members. This ruling cleared the obstacle that had prevented audiologists from competing directly with each other and with hearing instrument specialists. Although this change brought a whole new class of professionals to the hearing aid purchasing process, the hearing aid rule was not amended to incorporate this resource.

Although audiologists are not physicians and may not diagnose disease, their specialized university training prepares them to perform and interpret a wide variety of hearing-related tests as well as to recognize test results and patient symptoms that indicate the need for medical referral. Having professionals with this training begs the issue of whether a medical evaluation is necessary for the majority of people who are seen by an audiologist. A medical referral would certainly be given in the small percentage of cases in which history, symptoms, or test results point toward a medical problem. The majority of potential hearing aid candidates, however, might only need to make this one stop.

In addition, direct access to audiologists could allow for elimination of the existing medical waiver and in the process serve to improve consumer protection. All hearing aid candidates would be seen by an audiologist or physician (preferably one who specializes in ear problems). There would be no exceptions. Although it could be argued that an audiologist might overlook some obscure ear problem, the overall chance of this happening would seem much less than under the current system, in which many hearing aid candidates are seen by neither an audiologist or ear doctor. Hearing instrument specialists who follow the spirit of the current hearing aid rule would be largely unaffected since they would continue to obtain medical clearance for all their patients just as they always had. The end result would be a guaranteed minimum standard of care for everyone. There would be no more loopholes in the system. This is important not only from a standpoint of health but also for our next discussion.

Over-the-Counter Hearing Aids

Although the FDA regulates the hearing aid purchasing process, individual states can further regulate who may sell aids. A few retail or mail-order personal amplifiers of widely varying quality manage to slip between the regulatory cracks, but the vast majority of hearing aids are custom-made and dispensed by professionals. Despite all of the rules, regulations, medical concerns, audiologic justifications, special interests, and bureaucratic inertia that support the current dispensing system, many still wish low-cost over-the-counter (OTC) hearing aids were the norm rather than the exception.

At the same time that the petition was submitted to the FDA requesting the elimination of the medical clearance for hearing aids, a separate petition was submitted requesting approval for a new class of hearing aid (Killion 2003). This proposed one-size-fits-most hearing aid would be sold over the counter, without the requirement of a hearing test or medical examination. The petition argued that the people who suffer most under the current system are seniors on a fixed income, those without insurance benefits, and the poor. The creation of a readily accessible low-cost mass-produced hearing aid would end this de facto discrimination.

This petition was also denied by the FDA. The main stumbling block remained the issue of an examination before the purchase of hearing aids. Selling hearing aids over the counter without an examination left no safeguard for the public. The FDA did not want to go back to the days before the 1977 hearing aid rule (Boswell 2004).

Despite the FDA ruling, the issue of OTC hearing aids is not likely to go away. The need for some kind of low-cost hearing aid solution is too great. This issue was brought to the mainstream media in a *Wall Street Journal* report (Zimmerman 2004) titled "The Noisy Debate over Hearing Aids: Why So Expensive?" Although the article raised a number of important points, it tended to frame the issue as the defenseless public against the FDA and the big bad hearing aid people. Not surprisingly the article angered both sides. Much debate and name calling ensued, after which little was accomplished.

Obviously some middle ground is needed. Having the option to purchase a low-cost non-custom-made hearing aid is a good idea, but not if it risks the health of the public. What is needed is a way to rule out likely health concerns so that a lower-cost alternative can be available. One solution would be to require all potential hearing aid candidates to be evaluated by an ear doctor or audiologist. Once health issues are excluded, a person would then be free to choose the option that he or she prefers. A person could pursue the traditional course and buy custom-made hearing aids or purchase less expensive noncustom OTC aids. Although a noncustom aid would likely perform less effectively than one tailored specifically to an individual's needs, it might meet the individual's financial cost-to-hearing-benefit requirements. This approach is not likely to become reality, however, without public pressure for change.

If OTC hearing aids became a reality, the people most likely to benefit would be those with a mild or moderate hearing loss. Making sound loud enough to be heard yet not so loud as to be potentially damaging is readily achievable for this group, although it can be trickier when there is a more severe loss. Consequently OTC aids might not be the best option for more severe hearing losses. Because the majority of hearing losses fall within a mild or moderate range, making this option available after a medical or audiology examination would be a time and money saver for many.

In designing a one-size-fits-most hearing aid, a couple of the biggest challenges are fit and durability of the outer shell. The hard plastic or acrylic that would be the most durable is also the material most likely to cause discomfort if it rubs or presses against an ear. Softer materials that are more likely to be comfortable tend to wear out with use or are gradually broken down by earwax or a person's natural body oils. Solutions to these problems have recently been developed, but the products need to be mass-produced to become practical over-the-counter options. For example, the product Adesso was created by Sonic Innovations as a high-end digital hearing aid. The electronics of the aid were housed in a small, thin, CIC shell that was then covered with a changeable foam shell. The covering could be purchased in a thinner or thicker thickness that best fit an ear, and replacement shells could be purchased inexpensively as needed. Because of its small size, the aid was cosmetically pleasing. It was also comfortable to wear. Some people, however, objected to this one-size-fits-most aid because of how its high-end electronics and traditional dispensing affected cost. This particular model shows that practical solutions to potential fit problems with an OTC aid can be adopted by use of a model similar to Adesso but meant for a less affluent consumer. Another option might be using some form of small behind-the-ear aid with an open or extremely soft earmold design.

A final challenge for OTC hearing aids is that they currently lack the fine-tuning and individualization that is routine for professionally fit digital hearing aids. Even if an aid could be adjusted, the user does not have the tools or training to adjust the device correctly. Although this is a problem, it is not insurmountable. OTC hearing aids could be designed with an optional interface that would allow programming adjustments through a home computer. The wearer would enter his or her hearing test results into the computer, and user-friendly software would then program the hearing aid as well as guide the wearer through any later fine-tuning. Currently audiologists and hearing instrument specialists use sophisticated software that performs this task, and there is no reason that a safe, simple, and more intuitive version could not be developed for OTC aids. Another possibility might involve some form of wireless or Internet-based interface that programs the aid remotely. Although these over-the-counter options are still theoretical, they are options that may appeal to many and should be considered by the FDA and the general public. I hope baby boomers will one day benefit from cost-effective yet medically viable options such as these.

About Insurance

Government statistics place the number of Americans with no health insurance at 41 million or about 17 percent of the population (Schiller et al. 2005). For adults in late middle age—in other words baby boomers—the likelihood of being without health insurance at some point during the years preceding eligibility for Medicare is about 25 percent (Baker and Sudano 2005). By 2013, the number of uninsured is projected to rise to 56 million (Gilmer and Kronick 2005).

Cost is often the primary consideration when individuals or businesses select a health plan. Yet consumers should be aware that they're not choosing a low premium but sacrificing a lifetime of quality care. Insurance providers raise deductibles or limit benefits to reduce premiums. Consumers are well aware of the impact that deductibles can have on their budget but recognize this as a practical tradeoff against higher premiums. The issue of benefit reductions can be subtler. A provider may specifically exclude such "fringe" benefits as dental, vision, or hearing care. Another approach is to claim coverage for one or more of these "fringes" but to scale back the specifics of what is covered as to be nearly useless. Outright exclusion and hidden exclusion of specific services are issues to be aware of in selecting insurance coverage. Both are common with hearing care. With employer-provided insurance, of course, the choice of coverage has already been made for the employee.

As the baby boom generation continues to age, the problem of healthcare costs will only worsen. Most of the discussion about aging baby boomers focuses on how their large population will affect Social Security. The impact to Medicare will be equally problematic. The private sector had difficulty affording health insurance for baby boomers during their healthy working years. As boomers approach their senior years, this burden will soon be transferred to an already financially troubled public sector. It will be Medicare's responsibility to provide insurance for baby boomers that are now older and at even greater health risk. Unless something changes, it seems unlikely that Medicare will be able to provide insurance for the mass of aging baby boomers without having to follow the lead of the private sector and limiting benefits.

For there to be any hope that "ancillary" care benefits for hearing and vision will be available to baby boomers, Medicare will need to make heroic use of each healthcare dollar. Fortunately or unfortunately—depending on your viewpoint—it appears there is room for improvement. A report from the Cambridge Hospital and Harvard Medical School (Himmelstein et al. 2004) noted that "the United States wastes more on healthcare bureaucracy than it would cost to provide healthcare to all its uninsured." The authors calculated that administrative waste totaled $286 billion in 2003, or $6,940 that could have been applied toward healthcare for each of the 41.2 million uninsured. Who knew paper pushing could cost so much? Finding a way to eliminate this waste may well be the best chance for baby boomers to ensure their overall healthcare and hearing healthcare future.

You may feel powerless in the face of these grim statistics, but they are a call to action. They reinforce the importance of practicing hearing prevention now. They also suggest that you should plan financially for your own future hearing care. Setting aside a little extra money in a 401(k) or other pretax account is a good way to start.

Hearing Research

The importance of hearing research was briefly mentioned in the earlier discussion about nerve cell regeneration. If we truly want a better hearing aid or a cure for nerve hearing loss so that hearing aids may become unnecessary, serious research will likely be needed. Hearing aid manufacturers customarily fund their research through the sale of their existing products, but this is not a viable option for researchers with no product to sell. In the case of hearing aid research, there is little doubt that the product under development will have commercial value. In contrast, some of the most promising areas of hearing research such as nerve cell replacement or regeneration are highly speculative. They may change the world, but there is no guarantee of a marketable product. Consequently, research of this sort is not usually performed without outside funding.

The National Institutes of Health (NIH) is the best-known funding source for medical research. Funding levels for over two hundred diseases, conditions, and research areas are summarized on its website (NIH 2005). The categories range alphabetically from acute respiratory distress syndrome and Agent Orange to West Nile virus and women's health. The list details the money allocated for serious and well-recognized problems such as cancer and heart disease as well as for less life-threatening problems such as hay fever. Eye disease and vision disorders such as macular degeneration are on the list and reported to be well funded. Nowhere on the list, however, is hearing loss or ear disease. Only the ear infections that are most common in childhood (otitis media) made the cut. The omission of hearing loss does not mean that the NIH does not value or fund hearing research. It does, however, speak volumes about its assigned priority. Baby boomers need to be aware of this and find ways to make hearing loss a bigger concern. The criteria the NIH uses to determine research funding are highly complex, but it is likely that public interest, distress, and demand play at least a small role. The large population of baby boomers should be able to create the interest and demand before distress becomes the motivating factor.

One branch of the NIH that is extremely important in the area of hearing research is the National Institute on Deafness and Other Communication Disorders (NIDCD). It supports hundreds of ongoing research and education projects about hearing, balance, smell, taste, voice, and speech and language problems. Its website (http://www.nidcd.nih.gov) provides a wealth of information about hearing loss as well as updates on new and ongoing research. Although the NIDCD is federally funded, it accepts private contributions that can be earmarked for research. If you wish to donate money toward hearing research, this organization is a good one to contribute to.

Connecting the Dots

This book has provided a great deal of information about hearing loss, ear disease, medical treatments, hearing aids, and listening devices. After reading this book, baby boomers should recognize how hearing difficulties negatively impact many aspects of life. Approximately one in three baby boomers is likely to experience difficulty hearing firsthand within his or her lifetime. The remainder will experience it secondhand, through a spouse, friend, or co-worker. This secondhand exposure produces its own quality-of-life concerns.

Only once we recognize that hearing loss can affect us are we likely to act. Perhaps the biggest failing of past generations with regard to hearing loss is that they never had this realization. Even those who knew that hearing loss was a possibility did not usually seriously consider it before it became a problem. Consequently, they did little to prevent it, to educate themselves about it, or to demand that research be done in the area. The millions of people with noise-induced hearing loss are an end result of this oversight.

As baby boomers, we have the information needed to prevent or at least minimize the chance of developing hearing loss. If you already have a loss, you may be able to prevent it from worsening. Most importantly, avoid or protect yourself from loud noise. Turn down your stereo. Wear earplugs or muffs when operating power tools, chain saws, lawn tractors, or other loud tools. Always wear hearing protection while hunting. Make it convenient to protect your ears by leaving earplugs or earmuffs on or near loud sound sources so that they are always handy. I keep a set of noise-blocking earmuffs on the handle of my upright vacuum cleaner when it is not in use. In order to use the vacuum, I have to pick up the earmuffs to unwrap the power cord. I have another set of earmuffs hung within easy reach over my workbench. Taking steps such as these can dramatically increase the chance that you will make hearing protection a habit. Periodic hearing tests can then ensure that you are adequately protecting yourself or alert you if you need to do more.

If you suspect a hearing loss or know that you have one, get it checked. Denial and passivity are not good strategies in this area. The loss might be correctable, and you may be suffering needlessly. Even if it is not correctable, medical treatment or a change in behavior might keep it from getting worse. A slight loss caught early could remain slight rather than developing into a significant loss that cannot later be corrected.

Hearing aids are the best option for many people with hearing loss. This is true now and will likely remain so for some time to come. They greatly improve functionality, thereby eliminating many of the quality-of-life issues that hearing loss can produce. Although the individualized manufacturing, fitting, and programming process may lead to the best hearing, it also results in a high price tag. One challenge for baby boomers will be to decide whether the current hearing aid dispensing system should be left unchanged or whether there might be some practical lower-cost alternative. The final decision will likely involve a choice among safety, comfort, performance, and high cost versus economy. Any practical solution will lie somewhere between a high price tag and an inexpensive but less medically thorough alternative.

The whole subject of hearing care is most poignant when viewed in a personal rather than abstract way. Take a moment and consider your own situation by asking yourself a few questions. Do I have a hearing loss? Am I exposed to loud noise or other potential dangers to my ears? Should I be taking steps to preserve my hearing? Am I suffering a hearing loss without having checked to see if it might be treatable or even correctable? If it is not correctable, have I considered all the technological options for minimizing how the loss impacts me? Could or should I be taking an interest in hearing legislation or research from which I might ultimately benefit? Asking these questions is the first step to having a better hearing future. Acting on them is the second. It is my hope that you will be able to use the information in this book to do both. As a baby boomer, you not only owe yourself that opportunity but you have the time, resources, and strength in numbers to improve your hearing and also to improve national standards of hearing care for the better.

Resources

These resources are broadly categorized into associations, books, cochlear implants, hearing aids, magazines, and sources for assistive products. Inclusion in this list should not be considered an endorsement of any particular product or service. Similarly, omission from this list should not be construed negatively.

Associations

Alexander Graham Bell Association for the Deaf (AG Bell)
3417 Volta Place NW
Washington, DC 20007
Phone: 202-337-5220; TTY: 202-337-5221; fax: 202-337-8314
Website: www.agbell.org
E-mail: info@agbell.org
AG Bell is dedicated to promoting communication for people with
    hearing loss. It provides a support network and advocates for
    the hearing impaired.

American Academy of Audiology (AAA)
11730 Plaza America Dr., Suite 300
Reston, VA 20190
Phone: 800-222-2336: fax: 703-790-8631
Website: www.audiology.org
E-mail: form submitted from website.
AAA is the largest professional organization made up solely of audiolo-
    gists. The organization supports hearing care through advocacy,
    education, and research.

American Academy of Otolaryngology–Head and Neck Surgery
    (AAO-HNS)
1 Prince St.
Alexandria, VA 22314

Phone: 703-836-4444
Website: www.entnet.org
E-mail: form submitted from website.
The AAO-HNS is the world's largest organization of ear, nose, and
    throat physicians. Its website provides information on ear, nose,
    and throat disorders as well as a search engine for finding a physician
    in a particular area.

American Speech-Language-Hearing Association (ASHA)
10801 Rockville Pike
Rockville, MD 20852
Phone: 800-638-8255; TTY: 301-897-5700; fax: 301-571-0457
Website: www.asha.org
E-mail: actioncenter@asha.org
ASHA is the professional organization of over 100,000 speech-language
    pathologists, audiologists, and hearing scientists in the United States
    and internationally. Its website provides information on speech and
    hearing disorders as well as a search engine for finding a professional
    in a specific region.

American Tinnitus Association (ATA)
P.O. Box 5
Portland, OR 97207
Phone: 800-634-8978; fax: 503-248-0024
Website: www.ata.org
E-mail: tinnitus@ata.org
A perceived ringing, roaring, or cricket-like sound called tinnitus is
    common among people who have hearing loss. The ATA is possibly the
    best consumer source for information and support for this problem.

International Hearing Dog, Inc. (IHDI)
5901 E. 89th Ave.
Henderson, CO 80640
Phone/TTY: 303-287-3277; fax: 303-287-3425
Website: www.ihdi.org
E-mail: ihdi@aol.com
IHDI has trained hearing dogs for the deaf or hard of hearing since
    1979. The dogs are taught to alert a hearing-impaired person to a
    variety of sounds such as the doorbell or a smoke alarm. Mixed-breed
    dogs that have been saved from animal shelters are generally used.

League for the Hard of Hearing
50 Broadway, 6th floor
New York, NY 10004
Phone: 917-305-7700; TTY: 917-305-7999; fax: 917-305-7888
Website: www.lhh.org
E-mail: inf@lhh.org
The league's stated mission is to improve the quality of life of people
    with all degrees of hearing loss. In the nearly hundred years since it
    was founded, the League for the Hard of Hearing has helped over one
    million of the hearing impaired. It provides hearing and rehabilitative
    services regardless of age, mode of communication, or the ability
    to pay.

National Association of the Deaf (NAD)
814 Thayer Ave.
Silver Spring, MD 20910
Phone: 301-587-1788; TTY: 301-587-1789; fax: 301-587-1791
Website: www.nad.org
E-mail: nadinfo@nad.org
The NAD is a major advocate for the deaf and hard of hearing. It is
    a good source of information about the rights of hearing-impaired
    persons.

National Institute on Deafness and Other Communication Disorders
    (NIDCD)
National Institutes of Health
31 Center Dr., MSC 2320
Bethesda, MD 20892
Phone: 301-496-7243; TTY: 301-402-0252
Website: www.nidcd.nih.gov
E-mail: nidcdinfo@nidcd.nih.gov
The NIDCD, one of the institutes that make up the National Institutes
    of Health, supports behavioral and biomedical research related to
    hearing, balance, smell, taste, voice, and speech. Its website is an
    excellent source for information on ear and hearing disorders.

National Institutes of Health (NIH)
9000 Rockville Pike
Bethesda, MD 20892
Phone: 301-496-4000; TTY: 301-402-9612

Website: www.nih.gov

E-mail: nihinfo@od.nih.gov

The NIH is a part of the U.S. Department of Health and Human Services and is the primary federal funding agency for medical research. Its website provides a wealth of information on medical issues, including hearing loss, as well as an extensive list of links to other health resources.

Self Help for Hard of Hearing People (SHHH)

7910 Woodmont Ave., Suite 1200

Bethesda, MD 20814

Phone: 301-657-2248; TTY: 301-657-2249; fax: 301-913-9413

Website: www.shhh.org

E-mail: info@hearingloss.org

SHHH is the nation's largest organization for people with hearing loss. It provides education, information, and advocacy. SHHH has regional groups that form a national support network. Note: SHHH was renamed the Hearing Loss Association of America in March 2006.

Books

American Sign Language the Easy Way, by David Stewart (John Wiley and Sons)

This book, written for beginning American Sign Language (ASL) users, teaches the individual signs as well as ASL grammar and related information.

The Consumer Handbook on Hearing Loss and Hearing Aids: A Bridge to Healing, edited by Richard Carmen (Auricle Ink Publishers)

In this volume the editor brings together essays from a variety of hearing healthcare experts. It has been highly recommended by hearing professionals.

Living with Hearing Loss, by Marcia B. Dugan (Gallaudet University Press)

The author is a hearing loss sufferer and former president of Self Help for Hard of Hearing People. She provides some basics about hearing loss and suggestions for coping on a day-to-day basis.

Mayo Clinic on Hearing: Strategies for Managing Hearing Loss, Dizziness, and Other Ear Problems, by Wayne Olsen (Kensington Publishing Corporation)

This book covers a wide range of subjects, including the hearing examination, common hearing problems, treatment options, hearing aids, cochlear implants, tinnitus, and dizziness.

Overcoming Hearing Aid Fears: The Road to Better Hearing, by John M. Burkey (Rutgers University Press)
In this book I address common fears, concerns, and misconceptions that stand in the way of people purchasing and benefiting from hearing aids. Information is also presented about hearing aid styles, options, and costs.

A Quiet World: Living with Hearing Loss, by David Myers (Yale University Press)
The author shares his experience as a social psychologist and hearing loss sufferer. He explains the difficulties caused by hearing loss and gives advice on how to help a hearing-impaired loved one.

Speechreading: A Way to Improve Understanding, by Harriet Kaplan (Gallaudet University Press)
This volume is an at-home guide to learning speechreading (lipreading). Exercises are provided at the back of the book.

Wired for Sound: A Journey into Hearing, by Beverly Biderman (Trifolium Books)
This volume provides a personal account of living with a severe hearing loss and the difference a cochlear implant can make. This is a good resource for those trying to decide whether to have a cochlear implant.

Magazines

Hearing Health Magazine
Deafness Research Foundation
8201 Greensboro Dr., third floor
McLean, VA 22102
Phone: 800-829-5934; fax: 703-610-9005
Website: www.drf.org
E-mail: info@drf.org
Hearing Health Magazine is a publication of the Deafness Research Foundation. The magazine's goal is to keep readers informed of new research, treatments, and ways to cope with hearing loss.

Hearing Loss Magazine
Self Help for Hard of Hearing People (SHHH)
7910 Woodmont Ave., Suite 1200
Bethesda, MD 20814
Phone: 301-657-2248; TTY: 301-657-2249; fax: 301-913-9413
Website: www.hearingloss.org
E-mail: info@hearingloss.org
Hearing Loss Magazine is a publication of SHHH. It provides feature
 stories about hearing loss as well as information on research, treat-
 ment, and ways to cope with hearing impairment.

Cochlear Implants

Advanced Bionics
12740 San Fernando Rd.
Sylmar, CA 91342
Phone: 800-678-2575; TTY: 800-678-3575; fax: 661-362-1500
Website: www.bionicear.com
E-mail: info@advancedbionics.com
Advanced Bionics is the manufacturer of the Clarion and Bionic Ear
 multichannel cochlear implant systems. The company is well known
 and has a documented record of restoring sound to the severe and
 profoundly hearing impaired.

Cochlear Corporation
400 Inverness Parkway, Suite 400
Englewood, CO 80112
Phone/TTY: 800-523-5798; fax: 303-792-9025
Website: www.cochlear.com
E-mail: form submitted from website.
Cochlear Corporation has been at the forefront of cochlear implant
 research and development for over twenty-five years. Their Nucleus
 cochlear implant system has restored sound to many thousands of
 individuals worldwide.

Med-El Corporation
2222 E. NC Highway 54
Beta Bldg., Suite 180
Durham, NC 27713
Phone: 888-633-3524; TTY: 919-572-2222; fax: 919-454-9229
Website: www.medel.com

E-mail: implants@medelus.com

Med-El (Medical Electronics) Corporation is the other major player in
the field of cochlear implants. Similar to Cochlear Corporation and
Advanced Bionics, Med-El places a strong emphasis on research and
development. It has been responsible for a number of innovations
that are reflected in their product line.

Hearing Aids

Beltone
4201 West Victoria St.
Chicago, IL 60646
Phone: 800-621-1275
Website: www.beltone.com
E-mail: form submitted from website.

Beltone needs little introduction. The company has provided hearing
aids for over sixty years. This longevity, combined with extensive
consumer marketing, has made Beltone one of the most recognized
hearing aid brands.

Entific Medical Systems
7610 Olentangy River Dr., second floor
Columbus, OH 43235
Phone: 888-825-8484
Website: www.entific.com
E-mail: info@entificusa.com

Entific is the manufacturer of the Bone Anchored Hearing Aid System
(BAHA). The system consists of a small, externally worn sound
processor connected to a titanium fixture that has been surgically
implanted in the bone behind the ear. Sound is sent through the
fixture directly to the inner ear through bone conduction. The BAHA
is indicated for single-sided deafness and for conductive hearing
losses that are not medically correctable. Note: Cochlear Corporation
has recently acquired Entific, so the BAHA system may be listed with
them in the future. See Cochlear Corporation under cochlear
implants.

GN ReSound
8001 Bloomington Freeway
Bloomington, MN 55420
Phone: 800-248-4327

Website: www.gnresound.com
E-mail: form submitted from website.
GN ReSound is internationally known as an innovator. The company
was one of the early trendsetters in programmable and digital hearing
aid technology. It makes a full line of hearing aids and continues to
develop innovative new products.

Magnatone Hearing Aid Corp.
170 Cypress Way
Casselberry, FL 32707
Phone: 407-339-2422
Website: www.magnatone.com
E-mail: usa@magnatone.com
Magnatone has been manufacturing hearing aids for about forty
years. It is one of the few companies that offer a rechargeable
hearing aid.

Miracle Ear
5000 Cheshire Lane North
Plymouth, MN 55446
Phone: 888-283-9450
Website: www.miracle-ear.com
E-mail: form submitted from website.
Miracle Ear wins the award for best hearing aid name. This, combined
with its marketing, has made the brand well known. The company
has over one thousand centers across the United States and can be
found in many Sears department stores.

Oticon
29 Schoolhouse Rd.
Somerset, NJ 08873
Phone: 800-526-3921
Website: www.oticonus.com
E-mail: webmaster@oticonus.com
Founded in 1904, Oticon is one of the longest established hearing aid
manufacturers. Even after a hundred years, it remains a competitive
force in the hearing aid industry.

Phonak
4520 Weaver Parkway

Warrenville, IL 60555
Phone: 800-679-4871
Website: www.phonak-us.com
E-mail: info@phonak.com
Phonak makes several lines of hearing aids. Their BTE aids have earned
a reputation for durability among hearing professionals by standing
up to the abuse that is sometimes provided by hearing-impaired
children.

Phonic Ear
3880 Cypress Dr.
Petaluma, CA 94954
Phone: 800-227-0735
Website: www.phonicear.com
E-mail: customerservice@phonicear.com
Phonic Ear specializes in wireless systems for the hearing impaired.

Rexton
5010 Cheshire Lane North, Suite 2
Plymouth, MN 55446
Phone: 800-876-1141
Website: www.rexton.com
E-mail: form submitted from website.
Rexton has manufactured hearing aids for over forty years. Its hearing
aid designs have evolved with each technological advance, and it
continues to make an assortment of valued hearing aids.

Siemens Hearing Instruments
P.O. Box 1397
Piscataway, NJ 08855
Phone: 800-766-4500
Website: www.usa.siemens.com/hearing
E-mail: form submitted from website.
Siemens is a large multinational corporation and possibly the largest
manufacturer of hearing aids in the United States. It is committed
to research and manufactures a wide range of hearing aids and
hearing-related products.

Sonic Innovations
2795 E. Cottonwood Parkway, Suite 660

Salt Lake City, UT 84121
Phone: 888-678-4327
Website: www.sonici.com
E-mail: form submitted from website.
Sonic Innovations is one of the fastest growing hearing aid companies
    in the world. Its focus on digital technology has enabled it to
    develop a tiny digital signal processor that allows its hearing aids
    to physically fit into many small, narrow, or otherwise hard-to-fit
    ears.

Starkey Laboratories
6700 Washington Ave. South
Eden Prairie, MN 55344
Phone: 800-328-8602
Website: www.starkey.com
Starkey Laboratories has manufactured hearing aids for over thirty-five
    years. The company was an early supporter of a "trial" period in the
    hearing aid purchasing process. It was also one of the first to sell
    small CIC hearing aids. The Starkey Hearing Foundation, the com-
    pany's charitable organization, has provided hearing aids to thou-
    sands of people who could not otherwise afford them.

Unitron Hearing
2300 Berkshire Lane North
Plymouth, MN 55441
Phone: 800-888-8882
Website: www.unitronhearing.com
E-mail: info@unitronhearing.com
Unitron is another established and time-proven hearing aid
    manufacturer. It makes a full range of hearing aids, and its
    continuing research and development efforts keep its products
    competitive.

Widex Hearing Aid Company
35-53 24th St.
Long Island City, NY 11106
Phone: 800-221-0188
Website: www.widexusa.com
E-mail: form submitted from website.

Widex has manufactured hearing aids for over forty years. It makes several lines of high-end hearing aids and has been a consistent innovator in digital hearing aid technology.

Sources for Assistive Products

Harris Communications
15155 Technology Dr.
Eden Prairie, MN 55344
Phone: 800-825-6758; TTY: 800-825-9187; fax: 952-906-1099
Website: www.harriscomm.com
E-mail: info@harriscomm.com
Harris Communications sells a large selection of books, videos, telecommunication equipment, and assistive devices for the hearing impaired.

HITEC
8160 Madison Ave.
Burr Ridge, IL 60527
Phone: 800-288-8303; TTY: 800-536-8890
Website: www.hitec.com
E-mail: info@hitec.com
HITEC offers a wide variety of products for the hearing impaired, including devices for alerting and for assistive listening, as well as for telephone, television, and mobile communication.

LS&S Group Inc.
P.O. Box 673
Northbrook, IL 60065
Phone: 800-468-4789; TTY: 866-317-8533; fax: 847-498-1482
Website: www.lssproducts.com
E-mail: info@lssproducts.com
LS&S (Learning, Sight & Sound) Group has been serving the needs of the visually impaired and hard of hearing for over twenty years. Products range from Braille calculators to vibrating alarm clocks.

Sound Clarity
359 North 1st Ave.
Iowa City, IA 52245
Phone/TTY: 888-477-2995; fax: 319-354-5851

Website: www.soundclarity.com
E-mail: info@soundclarity.com
Sound Clarity provides an extensive array of hearing-related products. It sells alerting and assistive listening devices as well as amplified telephones and TTYs. It also sells pagers, hearing aid batteries, hearing protection, and less-sought-after items such as amplified stethoscopes.

References

American Academy of Otolaryngology–Head and Neck Surgery Foundation, Inc. 1982. *Guide for Conservation of Hearing in Noise*. Rev. ed. Rochester, MN.

American Association of Retired Persons [AARP]. 1994. *Aging Baby Boomers: How Secure Is Their Economic Future?* Washington, D.C.: AARP.

———. 2004. *Baby Boomers Envision Retirement II—Key Findings.* Washington, D.C.: AARP.

Arias, E. 2004. "United States Life Tables, 2001." In *National Vital Statistics Reports;* 52:14–44. Hyattsville, MD: National Center for Health Statistics.

Arias, E., R. N. Anderson, K. Hsiang-Ching, S. L. Murphy, and K. D. Kochanek. 2003. "Deaths: Final Data for 2001." In *National Vital Statistics Reports;* 52:3. Hyattsville, MD: National Center for Health Statistics.

Arkis P. N., and J. M. Burkey. 1994. "Word Recognition Scores: Do They Support Adaptation?" *Hearing Instruments* 45:24–25, 35.

Arlinger, S. 2003. "Negative Consequences of Uncorrected Hearing Loss—A Review." *International Journal of Audiology* 42 (2S):17–20.

Attias, J., G. Horovitz, N. El-Halib, and B. Nageris. 2001. "Detection and Clinical Diagnosis of Noise-Induced Hearing Loss by Otoacoustic Emissions." *Noise Health* 2 (12):19–31.

Attias, J., S. Sapir, I. Bresloff, I. Reshef-Haran, and H. Ising. 2004. "Reduction in Noise-Induced Temporary Threshold Shift in Humans following Oral Magnesium Intake." *Clinical Otolaryngology* 29 (6):635–641.

Attias, J., G. Weisz, S. Almog, A. Shahar, M. Wiener, Z. Joachims, A. Netzer, H. Ising, E. Rebentisch, and T. Guenther. 1994. "Oral Magnesium Intake Reduces Permanent Hearing Loss Induced by Noise Exposure." *American Journal of Otolaryngology* 15 (1):26–32.

Backous, D. D., N. J. Coker, and H. A. Jenkins. 1993. "Prospective Study of Resident-Performed Stapedectomy." *American Journal of Otology* 14 (5):451–454.

Baker D. W., and J. J. Sudano. 2005. "Health Insurance Coverage during the Years Preceding Medicare Eligibility." *Archives of Internal Medicine* 165 (7):770–776.

Bekesy, G. von. 1960. *Experiments in Hearing.* New York: McGraw-Hill.

Bentler, R. A., C. Palmer, and A. B. Dittberner. 2004. "Hearing-In-Noise: Comparison of Listeners with Normal and (Aided) Impaired Hearing." *Journal of the American Academy of Audiology* 15 (3):216–225.

Boswell, S. 2004. "FDA Rejects Citizen Petitions for Over-the-Counter Hearing Aids." *ASHA Leader,* April 27, pp. 1, 19.

Brant, L. J., S. Gordon-Salant, J. D. Pearson, L. L. Klein, C. H. Morrell, E. J. Metter, and J. L. Fozard. 1996. "Risk Factors Related to Age-Associated Hearing Loss in the Speech Frequencies." *Journal of the American Academy of Audiology* 7 (3):152–160.

Bray, A., M. Szmanski, and R. Mills. 2004. "Noise-Induced Hearing Loss in Dance Music Disc Jockeys and an Examination of Sound Levels in Nightclubs." *Journal of Laryngology and Otology* 118 (2):123–128.

Brookler, K. H., and H. Tanyeri. 1997. "Etidronate for the Neurotologic Symptoms of Otosclerosis: Preliminary Study." *Ear Nose and Throat Journal* 76 (6):371–376.

Brooks, D. N., R. S. Hallam, and P. A. Mellor. 2001. "The Effects on Significant Others of Providing a Hearing Aid to the Hearing-Impaired Partner." *British Journal of Audiology* 35:165–171.

Brownell, W.E. 1984. "Microscopic Observation of Cochlear Hair Cell Motility." *Scanning Electron Microscopy* 3:1401–6.

Brownell, W. E., C. R. Bader, D. Bertrand, and Y. Ribaupierre. 1985. "Evoked Mechanical Responses of Isolated Cochlear Outer Hair Cells." *Science* 227:194–196.

Burkey, J. M., and P. N. Arkis. 1993. "Word Recognition Changes after Monaural, Binaural Amplification." *Hearing Instruments* 44:8–9.

Byrne, D., H. Dillon, T. Ching, R. Katsch, and G. Keidser. 2001. "NAL-NL1 Procedure for Fitting Nonlinear Hearing Aids: Characteristics and Comparisons with Other Procedures." *Journal of the American Academy of Audiology* 12 (1):37–51.

Cacciatore, F., C. Napoli, P. Abete, E. Marciano, M. Triassi, and F. Rengo. 1999. "Quality of Life Determinants and Hearing Function in an Elderly Population: Osservatorio Geriatrico Campano Study Group." *Gerontology* 45 (6):323–328.

Camnitz, P. S., and W. S. Bost. 1985. "Traumatic Perforations of the Tympanic Membrane: Early Closure with Paper Tape Patching." *Otolaryngology Head and Neck Surgery* 93 (2):220–223.

Carhart, R. 1965. "Monaural and Binaural Discrimination against Competing Sentences." *International Journal of Audiology* 4:5–10.

Charasse, B., H. Thai-Van, J. M. Chanal, C. Berger-Vachon, and L. Collet. 2004. "Automatic Analysis of Auditory Nerve Electrically Evoked Compound Action Potential with an Artificial Neural Network." *Artificial Intelligence in Medicine* 31(3):221–229.

Chen, C. Y., C. Halpin, and S. D. Rauch. 2003. "Oral Steroid Treatment of Sudden Sensorineural Hearing Loss: A Ten-Year Retrospective Analysis." *Otology and Neurotology* 24 (5):728–733.

Chen, Z., M. Ulfendahl, R. Ruan, L. Tan, and M. Duan. 2004. "Protection of Auditory Function against Noise Trauma with Local Caroverine Administration in Guinea Pigs." *Hearing Research* 197(1–2):131–136.

Congressional Budget Office [CBO]. 2004. "The Retirement Prospects of the Baby Boomers." *Economic and Budget Issue Brief,* March 18, pp. 1–6.

Cord, M. T., M. R. Leek, and B. E. Walden. 2000. "Speech Recognition Ability in Noise and Its Relationship to Perceived Hearing Aid Benefit." *Journal of the American Academy of Audiology* 11 (9):475–483.

Cornelisse, L. E., R. C. Seewald, and D. G. Jamieson. 1995. "The Input/Output Formula: A Theoretical Approach to the Fitting of Personal Amplification Devices." *Journal of the Acoustical Society of America* 97(3):1854–1864.

Corwin, J. T., and D. A. Cotanche. 1988. "Regeneration of Sensory Hair Cells after Acoustic Trauma." *Science* 240:1772–1774.

Cotanche, D. A., 1987. "Regeneration of Hair Cell Stereociliary Bundles in the Chick Cochlea following Severe Acoustic Trauma." *Hearing Research* 30:181–196.

Cox, R. M. and G. C. Alexander. 2000. "Expectations about Hearing Aids and Their Relationship to Fitting Outcome." *Journal of the American Academy of Audiology* 11 (7):368–382.

———. 2001. "Validation of the SADL Questionnaire." *Ear and Hearing* 22 (2):151–160.

Cox, R. M., G. C. Alexander, and C. Gilmore. 1987. "Intelligibility of Average Talkers in Typical Listening Environments." *Journal of the Acoustical Society of America* 81 (5):1598–1608.

Cruickshanks, K. J., R. Klein, B. E. Klein, T. L. Wiley, D. M. Nondahl, and T. S. Tweed. 1998. "Cigarette Smoking and Hearing Loss: The Epidemiology of Hearing Loss Study." *Journal of the American Medical Association* 279 (21):1715–1719.

Cruickshanks, K. S., T. L. Wiley, T. S. Tweed, B. E. Klein, R. Klein, J. A. Mares-Perlman, and D. M. Nondahl. 1998. "Prevalence of Hearing

Loss in Older Adults in Beaver Dam, Wisconsin: The Epidemiology of Hearing Loss Study." *American Journal of Epidemiology* 148 (9): 879–886.

Cruz, R. M., P. R. Lambert, and E. W. Rubel. 1987. "Light Microscopic Evidence of Hair Cell Regeneration after Gentamicin Toxicity in the Chick Cochlea." *Archives of Otolaryngology Head and Neck Surgery* 113:1058–1062.

Dalton, D. S., K. J. Cruickshanks, B.E.K. Klein, R. Klein, T. L. Wiley, and D. M. Nondahl. 2003. "The Impact of Hearing Loss on Quality of Life in Older Adults." *Gerontologist* 5:661–668.

Dalton, D. S., K. J. Cruickshanks, T. L. Wiley, B. E. Klein, R. Kline, and T. S. Tweed. 2001. "Association of Leisure-Time Noise Exposure and Hearing Loss." *Audiology* 40 (1):1–9.

Dent, H. S. 2004. *The Next Great Bubble Boom: How to Profit from the Greatest Boom in History, 2005–2009.* New York: Free Press.

Dermody, P., and D. Byrne. 1975. "Loudness Summation with Binaural Hearing Aids." *Scandinavian Audiology* 4:23–28.

Desai, M., L. A. Pratt, H. Lentzner, and K. N. Robinson. 2001. "Trends in Vision and Hearing among Older Americans." *Aging Trends* 2:1–8.

Di Nardo, W., S. Ippolito, N. Quaranta, G. Cadoni, and J. Galli. 2003. "Correlation between NRT Measurement and Behavioral Levels in Patients with the Nucleus 24 Cochlear Implant." *Acta Otorhinolaryngologica Italica* 23 (5):352–355.

Divenyi, P. L., and K. M. Haupt. 1997. "Audiological Correlates of Speech Understanding Deficits in Elderly Listeners with Mild-to-Moderate Hearing Loss. III. Factor Representation." *Ear and Hearing* 18 (3): 189–201.

Duan, M., J. Qiu, G. Laurell, A. Ologsson, S. A. Counter, and E. Borg. 2004. "Dose and Time-Dependent Protection of the Antioxidant N-L-Acetylcysteine against Impulse Noise Trauma." *Hearing Research* 192 (1–2):1–9.

Dyrlund, O., and N. Bisgaard. 1991. "Acoustic Feedback Margin Improvements in Hearing Instruments Using a Prototype DFS (Digital Feedback Suppression) System." *Scandinavian Audiology* 20 (1):49–53.

Dyrlund, O., L. B. Henningsen, N. Bisgaard, and J. H. Jensen. 1994. "Digital Feedback Suppression (DFS): Characterization of Feedback-Margin Improvements in a DFS Hearing Instrument." *Scandinavian Audiology* 23 (2):135–138.

Emmer. M. 1990. "The Effect of Lack of Amplification on Speech Recognition in the Unaided Ear." *Hearing Instruments* 41:16.

Faiers, F., and P. McCarthy. 2004. "Study Explores How Paying Affects Hearing Aid Users' Satisfaction." *Hearing Journal* 57 (12):25–32.

Flemming, N. 1939. "Resonance of the External Auditory Meatus." *Nature* 143:642–643.

Florentine, M., W. Hunter, M. Robinson, M. Ballou, and S. Buss. 1998. "On the Behavioral Characteristics of Loud-Music Listening." *Ear and Hearing* 19 (6):420–428.

Gale, W. G. 1997. "The Aging of America: Will the Baby Boom Be Ready for Retirement?" *Brookings Review* 15 (3):4–9.

Garcia Callejo, F. J., J. Marco Algarra, M. P. Martinez Beneyto, M. H. Orts Alborch, and A. Morant Ventura. 2003. "Autoimmune Identification of Sudden Hearing Loss." *Acta Otolaryngologica* 123 (2):168–171.

Gates, G. A., J. L. Cobb, R. B. D'Agostino, and P. A. Wolfe. 1993. "The Relation of Hearing in the Elderly to the Presence of Cardiovascular Disease and Cardiovascular Risk Factors." *Archives of Otolaryngology Head and Neck Surgery* 119:156–161.

Gelfand, S. A. 1995. "Long-Term Recovery and No Recovery from the Auditory Deprivation Effect with Binaural Amplification: Six Cases." *Journal of the American Academy of Audiology* 6:141–149.

Gelfand, S., S. Silman, and L. Ross. 1989. "Long-Term Effects of Monaural, Binaural and No Amplification in Subjects with Bilateral Hearing Loss." *Scandinavian Audiology* 16:201–207.

General Accounting Office. 2002. *Long-Term Care: Aging Baby Boom Generation Will Increase Demand and Burden on Federal and State Budgets* GAO-02-544T. Washington, DC.

Gill, T. M., and A. R. Feinstein. 1994. "A Critical Appraisal of the Quality of Quality-of-Life Measurements." *Journal of the American Medical Association* 272:619–626.

Gilmer, T., and R. Kronick. 2005. "It's the Premiums, Stupid: Projections of the Uninsured Through 2013." *Health Affairs* [E-pub ahead of print].

Girod, D. A., L. G. Duckert, and E. W. Rubel. 1989. "Possible Precursors of Regenerated Hair Cells in the Avian Cochlea Following Acoustic Trauma." *Hearing Research* 42:175–194.

Gist, J.R., K. D. Wu, and C. Ford. 1999. "Do Baby Boomers Save and, If So, What For?" Publication number 9906. Washington, DC.

Golz, A., D. Goldenberg, A. Netzer, M. Fradis, S. T. Westerman, L. M. Westerman, and H. Z. Joachims. 2003. "Paper Patching for Chronic Tympanic Membrane Perforations." *Otolaryngology Head and Neck Surgery* 128 (4):565–570.

Gratton, M. A., and A. E. Vazquez. 2003. "Age-Related Hearing Loss: Current Research." *Current Opinions in Otolaryngology Head and Neck Surgery* 11 (5):367–371.

Gudmundsen, G. 2003. Citizen petition. FDA docket no. 2003P–0363.

Hamzavi, J., P. Franz, W. D. Baumgartner, and W. Gostettner. 2001. "Hearing Performance in Noise of Cochlear Implant Patients versus Severely-Profoundly Hearing-Impaired Patients with Hearing Aids." *Audiology* 40 (1):26–31.

Harris, R. W., and M. L. Reitz. 1985. "Effects of Room Reverberation and Noise on Speech Discrimination by the Elderly." *Audiology* 24 (5):319–324.

Helfer, K. S., and R. L. Freyman. 2005. "The Role of Visual Speech Cues in Reducing Energetic and Informational Masking." *Journal of the Acoustical Society of America* 117 (2):842–849.

Hetu, R., and M. Fortin. 1995. "Potential Risk of Hearing Damage Associated with Exposure to Highly Amplified Music." *Journal of the American Academy of Audiology* 6 (5):378–386.

Heine, C., and C. J. Browning. 2002. "Communication and Psychosocial Consequences of Sensory Loss in Older Adults: Overview and Rehabilitation Directions." *Disability and Rehabilitation* 24:763–773.

Higgins, K. M., J. M. Chen, J. M. Nedzelski, D. B. Shipp, and L. D. McIlmoyl. 2002. "A Matched-Pair Comparison of Two Cochlear Implant Systems." *Journal of Otolaryngology* 31 (2):97–105.

Hight, N. G., S. L. McFadden, D. Henderson, R. F. Burkard, and T. Nicotera. 2003. "Noise-Induced Hearing Loss in Chinchillas Pre-Treated with Glutathione Monoethylester and R-PIA." *Hearing Research* 179 (1–2):21–32.

Himmelstein, D. U., S. Woolhandler, and S .M. Wolfe. 2004. "Administrative Waste in the U.S. Healthcare System in 2003: The Cost to the Nation, the States, and the District of Columbia, with State-Specific Estimates of Potential Savings." *International Journal of Health Services* 34 (1):79–86.

Hu, Z., D. Wei, C. B. Johansson, N. Holmstrom, M. Duan, J. Frisen, and M. Ulfendahl. 2005. "Survival and Neural Differentiation of Adult Neural Stem Cells Transplanted into the Mature Inner Ear." *Experimental Cell Research* 302 (1):40–47.

Hughes, G. B. 1991. "The Learning Curve in Stapedectomy." *Laryngoscope* 101 (12):1280–1284.

Itoh, A., T. Nakashima, H. Arao, K. Wakai, A. Tamakoshi, T. Kawamura, and Y. Ohno. 2001. "Smoking and Drinking Habits as Risk Factors for

Hearing Loss in the Elderly: Epidemiological Study of Subjects Undergoing Routine Health Checks in Aichi, Japan." *Public Health* 115 (3):192–196.

Izumikawa, M., R. Minoda, K. Kawamoto, K. A. Abrashkin, D. L. Swiderski, D. F. Dolan, D. E. Brough, and Y. Raphael. 2005. "Auditory Hair Cell Replacement and Hearing Improvement by Atoh1 Gene Therapy in Deaf Mammals." *Nature Medicine* 11 (3):271–276.

Jerram, J. C., and S. C. Purdy. 2001. "Technology, Expectations, and Adjustment to Hearing Loss: Predictors of Hearing Aid Outcome." *Journal of the American Academy of Audiology* 12 (2):64–79.

Jones, L. Y. 1980. *Great Expectations: America and the Baby Boom Generation.* New York: Ballantine Books.

Joson, H. A., F. Asano, Y. Suzuki, and T. Sone. 1993. "Adaptive Feedback Cancellation with Frequency Compression for Hearing Aids." *Journal of the Acoustical Society of* America 94 (6):3254–3258.

Kakarlapudi, V., R. Sawyer, and H. Staicker. 2003. "The Effect of Diabetes on Sensorineural Hearing Loss." *Otology and Neurotology* 24 (3):382–386.

Kawamoto, K., S. Ishimoto, R. Minoda, D. E. Brough, and Y. Raphael. 2003. "Math1 Gene Transfer Generates New Cochlear Hair Cells in Mature Guinea Pigs in Vivo." *Journal of Neuroscience* 23(11):4395–4400.

Keidser, G. 1995. "The Relationship between Listening Conditions and Alternative Amplification Schemes for Multiple Memory Hearing Aids." *Ear and Hearing* 16 (6):575–586.

Kemp, D. T. 1978. "Stimulated Acoustic Emissions from within the Human Auditory System." *Journal of the Acoustical Society of America* 64:1386–1391.

———. 1979. "Evidence of Mechanical Nonlinearity and Frequency Selective Wave Amplification in the Cochlea." *Archives of Otorhinolaryngology* 224:37–45.

Kemp, M. 1998. "Why is Learning American Sign Language a Challenge?" *American Annals of the Deaf* 143 (3):255–259.

Killion, M. 2003. Citizen petition. FDA docket no. 2003P–0362.

Kiss, J. G., F. Toth, A. L. Nagy, J. Jarabin, A. Szamoskozi, J. Torkos, J. Jori, and J. Czigner. 2003. "Neural Response Telemetry in Cochlear Implant Users." *International Tinnitus Journal* 9 (1):59–60.

Kochkin, S. 1993. "MarkeTrak III: Higher Hearing Aid Sales Don't Signal Better Market Penetration." *Hearing Journal* 46 (7):47–54.

———. 1994. "MarkeTrak IV: Impact on Purchase Intent of Cosmetics, Stigma, and Style of Hearing Instrument." *Hearing Journal* 47 (9): 29–36.

————. 1996. "MarkeTrak IV: Ten-Year Trends in the Hearing Aid Market: Has Anything Changed?" *Hearing Journal* 48 (1):23–34.

————. 2001. "The VA and Direct Mail Sales Spark Growth in Hearing Aid Market." *Hearing Review* 8:16–24, 63–65.

————. 2002. "MarkeTrak VI: 10-Year Customer Satisfaction Trends in the U.S. Hearing Instrument Market." *Hearing Review* 9 (10):14–25;46.

————. 2003a. "MarkeTrak VI: On the Issue of Value: Hearing Aid Benefit, Price, Satisfaction, and Brand Repurchase Rates." *Hearing Review* 10 (2):12–26.

————. 2003b. "MarkeTrak VI: Isolating the Impact of the Volume Control on Customer Satisfaction." *Hearing Review* 10 (1):26–35.

Kramer, S. E., T. S. Kapteyn, D. J. Kuik, and D.J.H. Deeg. 2002. "The Association of Hearing Impairment and Chronic Diseases with Psychological Health Status on Older Age." *Journal of Aging and Health* 14:122–137.

Kubler-Ross, E. 1969. *On Death and Dying*. New York: Macmillan.

Lamden, K. H., A. S. St Leger, and J. Raveglia. 1995. "Hearing Aids: Value for Money and Health Gain." *Journal of Public Health Medicine* 17 (4):445–449.

Lapsley Miller, J. A., L. Marshall, and L. M. Heller. 2004. "A Longitudinal Study of Changes in Evoked Otoacoustic Emissions and Pure-Tone Thresholds as Measured in a Hearing Conservation Program." *International Journal of Audiology* 43 (6):307–322.

Larson, V. D., D. W. Williams, W. G. Henderson, L. E. Luethke, L. B. Beck, D. Noffsinger, G. W. Bratt, R. A. Dobie, S. A. Fausti, G. B. Haskell, B. Z. Rappaport, J. E. Shanks, and R. H. Wilson. 2002. "A Multi-Center, Double-Blind Clinical Trial Comparing Benefit from Three Commonly Used Hearing Aid Circuits." *Ear and Hearing* 23 (4):269–276.

Latzel, M., T. M. Gebhart, and J. Kiessling. 2001. "Benefit of a Digital Feedback Suppression System for Acoustical Telephone Communication." *Scandinavian Audiology* (suppl.) 52:69–72.

Lippy, W. H., R. A. Battista, L. Berenholz, A. G. Schuring, and J. M. Burkey. 2003. "Twenty-Year Review of Revision Stapedectomy." *Otology and Neurotology* 24 (4):560–566.

Lippy, W. H., J. M. Burkey, M. J. Fucci, A. G. Schuring, and F. M. Rizer. 1996. "Stapedectomy in the Elderly." *American Journal of Otology* 17:831–834.

Lucertini, M., A. Moleti, and R. Sisto. 2002. "On the Detection of Early Cochlear Damage by Otoacoustic Emission Analysis." *Journal of the Acoustical Society of America* 111 (2):972–978.

Lustig, L. R., H. A. Arts, D. E. Brackmann, H. F. Francis, T. Molony, C. A. Megerian, G. F. Moore, K. M. Moore, T. Morrow, W. Potsic, J. T. Rubenstein, S. Srireddy, C. A. Syms, G. Takahashi, D. Vernick, P. A. Wackym, and J. K. Niparko. 2001. "Hearing Rehabilitation Using the BAHA Bone-Anchored Hearing Aid: Results in 40 Patients." *Otology and Neurotology* 22 (3):328–334.

Marean, G. C., J. M. Burt, M. D. Beecher, and E. W. Rubel. 1993. "Hair Cell Regeneration in the Starling (*Sturnus vulgaris*): Recovery of Pure-Tone Detection Thresholds." *Hearing Research* 71(1–2):125–136.

Martin, J. A., B. E. Hamilton, S. J. Ventura, F. Menacker, M. M. Park, and P. D. Sutton. 2002. "Births: Final Data for 2001." In *National Vital Statistics Reports* 51:2. Hyattsville, MD: National Center for Statistics.

Meister, H., I. Lausberg, J. Kiessling, H. von Wedel, and M. Walger. 2004. "Detecting Components of Hearing aid Fitting Using a Self-Assessment-Inventory." *European Archives of Otorhinolaryngology* [E-pub ahead of print].

Meyer T. T., and P. R. Lambert. 2004. "Primary and Revision Stapedectomy in Elderly Patients." *Current Opinions in Otolaryngology Head and Neck Surgery* 12 (5):387–392.

Meyer-Bisch, C. 1996. "Epidemiological Evaluation of Hearing Damage Related to Strongly Amplified Music (Personal Cassette Players, Discotheques, Rock Concerts) High-Definition Audiometric Survey on 1364 Subjects." *Audiology* 35 (3):121–142.

Mo, B., M. Lindbaek, and S. Harris. 2005. "Cochlear Implants and Quality of Life: A Prospective Study." *Ear and Hearing* 26 (2):186–194.

Morata T. C., and M. B. Little. 2002. "Suggested Guidelines for Studying the Combined Effects of Occupational Exposure to Noise and Chemicals on Hearing." *Noise Health* 4 (14):73–87.

Mulrow, C. D., C. Aguilar, J. E. Endicott, R. Velez, M. R. Tuley, W. S. Charlip, and J. A. Hill. 1990. "Association between Hearing Impairment and the Quality of Life of Elderly Individuals." *Journal of the American Geriatric Society* 38:45–50.

Mulrow, C. D., M. R. Tuley, and C. Aguilar. 1992. "Sustained Benefits of Hearing Aids." *Journal of Speech and Hearing Research* 35 (6):1402–1405.

Nabelek, A. K., J. W. Tampas, and S. B. Burchfield. 2004. "Comparison of Speech Perception in Background Noise with Acceptance of Background Noise in Aided and Unaided Conditions." *Journal of Speech, Language and Hearing Research* 47 (5):1001–1011.

National Council on Aging. 2000. "The Consequences of Untreated Hearing Loss in Older Persons." *Otorhinolaryngology Head and Neck Nursing* 18, 1 (Winter):12–16.

National Institute on Deafness and Other Communication Disorders. 1989. *A Report on the Task Force on the National Strategic Plan.* Bethesda, MD: National Institutes of Health.

National Institutes of Health [NIH]. 2005. *Estimates of Funding for Various Diseases, Conditions, Research Areas.* As listed on NIH website: *http://www.nih.gov/news/fundingresearchareas.htm* Updated March 8, 2005.

Needleman, A. R., and C. C. Crandell. 1995. "Speech Recognition in Noise by Hearing-Impaired and Noise-Masked Normal-Hearing Listeners." *Journal of the American Academy of Audiology* 6 (6):414–424.

Noffsinger, D., G. B. Haskell, V. D. Larson, D. W. Williams, E. Wilson, S. Plunkett, and D. Kenworthy. 2002. "Quality Rating Test of Hearing Aid Benefit in the NIDCD/VA Clinical Trial." *Ear and Hearing* 23 (4): 291–300.

Nondahl, D. M., K. J. Cruickshanks, T. L. Wiley, R. Klein, and T. S. Tweed. 2000. "Recreational Firearm Use and Hearing Loss." *Archives of Family Medicine* 9 (4):352–357.

Palmer, K. T., M .J. Griffin, H. E. Syddall, and D. Coggon. 2004. "Cigarette Smoking, Occupational Exposure to Noise, and Self-Reported Hearing Difficulties." *Occupational Environmental Medicine* 61 (4):340–344.

Pasanisi, E., A. Bacciu, V. Vincenti, M. Guida, A. Barbot, M. T. Berghenti, and S. Bacciu. 2003. "Speech Recognition in Elderly Cochlear Implant Recipients." *Clinical Otolaryngology* 28 (2):154–157.

Physicians' Desk Reference. 2004. Montvale, NJ: Thompson PDR.

Pirodda, A., G. G. Rerri, G. C. Modugno, and A. Gaddi. 1999. "Hypotension and Sensorineural Hearing Loss: A Possible Correlation." *Acta Otolaryngologica* 119 (7):758–762.

Plakke, B. L. and E. Dare. 1992. "Occupational Hearing Loss in Farmers." *Public Health Reports* 107 (2):188–192.

Pourbakht, A., and T. Yamasoba. 2003. "Ebselen Attenuates Cochlear Damage Caused by Acoustic Trauma." *Hearing Research* 181 (1–2):100–108.

Puls, T. 1997. "Stapes Surgery: Results When Performing a Moderate Number of Stapedectomies." *Acta Otorhinolaryngologica Belgium* 51 (1):23–25.

Ricketts, T., P. Henry, and D. Gnewikow. 2003. "Full-Time Directional versus User Selectable Microphone Modes in Hearing Aids." *Ear and Hearing* 34 (5):424–439.

Ricketts, T, and H. G. Mueller. 2000. "Predicting Directional Hearing Aid Benefit for Individual Listeners." *Journal of the American Academy of Audiology* 11 (10):561–569.

Ries, P. W. 1994. "Prevalence and Characteristics of Persons with Hearing Trouble: United States, 1990–91." National Health Survey Series 10, no. 188.

Rizer, F. M. 1997a. "Overlay Versus Underlay Tympanoplasty. Part I: Historical Review of the Literature." *Laryngoscope* 107 (suppl. 84):1–25.

———. 1997b. "Overlay Versus Underlay Tympanoplasty. Part II: The Study." *Laryngoscope* 107 (suppl. 84):26–36.

Rizer, F. M., and W. H. Lippy. 1993. "Evolution of Techniques of Stapedectomy from the Total Stapedectomy to the Small Fenestra Stapedectomy." *Otolaryngologic Clinics of North America* 26 (3):443–451.

Roland, J. T. 2000. "Autoimmune Inner Ear Disease." *Current Rheumatology Reports* 2 (2):171–174.

Ruckenstein, M. J. 2004. "Autoimmune Inner Ear Disease." *Current Opinions in Otolaryngology Head and Neck Surgery* 12(5):426–430.

Ryals, B. M., and E. W. Rubel. 1988. "Hair Cell Regeneration after Acoustic Trauma in Adult Coturnix Quail." *Science* 240:1774–1776.

Rybak, L. P. 1992. "Hearing: The Effects of Chemicals." *Otolaryngology Head and Neck Surgery* 106:677–686.

Sargent, E. W. 2002. "The Learning Curve Revisited: Stapedectomy." *Otolaryngology Head and Neck Surgery* 126 (1):20–25.

Scheibe, F., H. Haupt, B. Mazurek, and O. Konig. 2001. "Therapeutic Effect of Magnesium on Noise-Induced Hearing Loss." *Noise Health* 3 (11):79–84.

Scherer, M. J., and D. R. Frisina. 1998. "Characteristics Associated with Marginal Hearing Loss and Subjective Well-Being among a Sample of Older Adults." *Journal of Rehabilitation Research and Development* 35:420–426.

Schiller, J. S., P. F. Adams, and Z. C. Nelson. 2005. "Summary Health Statistics for the U.S. Population: National Health Interview Survey, 2003." *Vital Health Statistics* 10 (224):1–104.

Schum, D. G. 1999. "Perceived Hearing Aid Benefit in Relation to Perceived Needs." *Journal of the American Academy of Audiology* 10 (1):40–45.

Schuring, A. G., and W. H. Lippy. 1985. "Validating the Excision of Cholesteatoma." *Otolaryngology Head and Neck Surgery* 93 (3):288–292.

Schuring, A. G., W. H. Lippy, F. M. Rizer, and L. T. Schuring. 1990. "Staging for Cholesteatoma in the Child, Adolescent, and Adult." *Annals Otology, Rhinology and Laryngology* 99 (4):256–260.

Seixas, N. S., S. G. Kujawa, S. Norton, L. Sheppard, R. Neitzel, and A. Slee. 2004. "Predictors of Hearing Threshold Levels and Distortion Product Otoacoustic Emissions among Noise-Exposed Young Adults." *Occupational Environmental Medicine* 61 (11):899–907.

Shambaugh, G. E., Jr. 1989. "How and When to Prescribe Sodium Fluoride." *American Journal of Otology* 10 (2):146–147.

Sharabi, Y., I. Reshef-Haran, M. Burstein, and A. Eldad. 2002. "Cigarette Smoking and Hearing Loss: Lessons from the Young Adult Periodic Examinations in Israel (YAPEIS) Database." *Israel Medical Association Journal* 4 (12):1118–1120.

Shea, J. J., Jr. 1998. "Forty Years of Stapes Surgery." *American Journal of Otology* 19 (1):52–55.

Shearer, P. D. 1990. "The Deafness of Beethoven: An Audiologic and Medical Overview." *American Journal of Otology* 11 (5):370–374.

Shou, J., J. L Zheng, and W. Q. Gao. 2003. "Robust Generation of New Hair Cells in the Mature Mammalian Inner Ear by Adenoviral Expression of Hath1." *Molecular and Cellular Neurosciences* 23 (2):169–179.

Siegel, J. 1996. "Aging into the 21st Century." Washington, DC: Department of Health and Human Services Administration on Aging.

Silman, S., S. Gelfand, and C. Silverman. 1984. "Late-Onset Auditory Deprivation: Effects on Monaural versus Binaural Hearing Aids." *Journal of the Acoustical Society of America* 76:1357–1362.

Silverman, C. A., and M. B. Emmer. 1993. "Auditory Deprivation and Recovery in Adults with Asymmetric Sensorineural Hearing Impairment." *Journal of the American Academy of Audiology* 4:338–346.

Slattery, W. H., L. M. Fisher, Z. Iqbal, and N. Liu. 2005. "Oral Steroid Regimens for Idiopathic Sudden Sensorineural Hearing Loss." *Otolaryngology Head and Neck Surgery* 132 (1):5–10.

Sliwinska-Kowalska, M. E., W. Zamyslowska-Szmytke, P. Szymczak, M. Kotlo, M. Fiszer, W. Wesolowski, and M. Pawlaczyk-Luszczynska. 2003. "Ototoxic Effects of Occupational Exposure to Styrene and Co-Exposure to Styrene and Noise." *Journal of Occupational Environmental Medicine* 45 (1):15–24.

Stahle, J. 1984. "Medical Treatment of Fluctuant Hearing Loss in Meniere's Disease." *American Journal of Otology* 5 (6): 529–533.

Stangerup, S. E., M. Tos, P. Caye-Thomasen, T. Tos, M. Klokker, and J. Thomsen. 2004. "Increased Annual Incidence of Vestibular Schwannoma and Age at Diagnosis." *Journal of Laryngology and Otology* 118 (4):622–627.

Stark, P., and L. Hickson. 2004. "Outcomes of Hearing Aid Fitting for Older People with Hearing Impairment and Their Significant Others." *International Journal of Audiology* 43 (7):390–398.

Stephens, D., L. France, and K. Lormore. 1995. "Effects of Hearing Impairment on the Patient's Family and Friends." *Acta Otolaryngologica* 115:165–167.

Strom, K. E. 2004. "The HR 2004 Dispenser Survey." *Hearing Review* 11 (6):14–32, 58–59.

———. 2005. "The HR 2005 Dispenser Survey." *Hearing Review* 12 (6):18–36, 72.

Surr, R. K., M. T. Cord, and B. E. Walden. 2001. "Response of Hearing Aid Wearers to the Absence of a User-Operated Volume Control." *Hearing Journal* 54 (4):32–36.

Talbott, E. O., R. C. Findlay, L. H. Kuller, L. A. Lenkner, K. A. Matthews, R. D. Day, and E. K. Ishii. 1990. "Noise-Induced Hearing Loss: A Possible Marker for High Blood Pressure in Older Noise-Exposed Populations." *Journal of Occupational Medicine* 32 (8):690–697.

Tateya, I., T. Nakagawa, F. Iguchi, T. S. Kim, T. Endo, S. Yamada, R. Kageyama, Y. Naito, and J. Ito. 2003. "Fate of Neural Stem Cells Grafted into Injured Inner Ears of Mice." *Neuroreport* 14 (13):1677–1681.

Texas Department on Aging. 2000. *The Texas Baby Boomer Survey.* Austin, TX.

Tucci, D. L., and E. W. Rubel. 1990. "Physiological Status of Regenerated Hair Cells in the Avian Inner Ear Following Aminoglycoside Ototoxicity." *Otolaryngology Head and Neck Surgery* 103:443–450.

United States v. National Society of Professional Engineers, No. 76–1767. 1978. *American Speech Language and Hearing Association* 20: 542–549.

U.S. Census Bureau. 2000. *Educational Attainment of the Population 15 Years and Over, by Age, Sex, Race and Hispanic Origin.* Washington DC.

U.S. Congress. 1990. *Americans with Disabilities Act of 1990.* Public Law 101–336. Washington DC.

U.S. Department of Labor. 1989. *Occupational Noise Exposure.* 29 CFR (1910.95):179–193. Washington, DC.

U.S. Food and Drug Administration. 1977. *Subpart H—Special Requirements for Specific Devices: Conditions for Hearing Aid Devices.* 21CFR801.421. Washington, DC.

Vesterager, V., G. Salomon, and M. Jagd. 1988. "Age-Related Hearing Difficulties." *Audiology* 27:179–192.

Vital and Health Statistics. 1964. "Natality Statistics Analysis: United States—1962." Washington, DC: National Center for Health Statistics.

Walden, B. E., R. K. Surr, M. T. Cord, B. Edwards, and l. Olson. 2000. "Comparison of Benefits Provided by Different Hearing Aid Technologies." *Journal of the American Academy of Audiology* 11 (10):540–560.

Walden, T. C., and B. E. Walden. 2004. "Predicting Success with Hearing Aids in Everyday Living." *Journal of the American Academy of Audiology* 15 (5):342–352.

Wallhagen, M. I., W. J. Strawbridge, R. D. Cohen, and G. A. Kaplan. 1997. "An Increasing Prevalence of Hearing Impairment and Associated Factors over Three Decades of the Alameda County Study." *American Journal of Public Health* 87 (3):333–334.

Wallhagen, M. I., W .J. Strawbridge, S. J. Shema, and G. A. Kaplan. 2004. "Impact of Self-Assessed Hearing Loss on a Spouse: A Longitudinal Analysis of Couples." *Journal of Gerontology Series B: Psychological Sciences and Social Sciences* 59:S190–196.

Walsh-Healey Public Contracts Act. 1969. *Federal Register* 34, no. 96. Washington, DC.

Wazen, J. J., J. B. Spitzer, S. N. Ghossaini, J. N. Fayad, J. K. Niparko, K. Cox, D. E. Brackmann, and S. D. Soli. 2003. "Transcranial Contralateral Cochlear Stimulation in Unilateral Deafness." *Otolaryngology Head and Neck Surgery* 129 (3):248–254.

Wazen, J. J., J. B. Spitzer, S. N. Ghossaini, A. Kacker, and A. Zschommler. 2001. "Results of the Bone-Anchored Hearing Aid in Unilateral Hearing Loss." *Laryngoscope* 111 (6):955–958.

Weinstein, B. E. 1996. "Treatment Efficacy: Hearing Aids in the Management of Hearing Loss in Adults." *Journal of Speech and Hearing Research* 39:S37–45.

Wiley, T. L., K. J. Cruickshanks, D. M. Nondahl, and T. S. Tweed. 2000. "Self-Reported Hearing Handicap and Audiometric Measures in Older Adults." *Journal of the American Academy of Audiology* 11:67–75.

Wilson, R. H. 2003. "Development of a Speech-in-Multitalker-Babble Paradigm to Assess Word-Recognition Performance." *Journal of the American Academy of Audiology* 14 (9):453–470.

Wilson, W. J., and N. Herbstein. 2003. "The Role of Music Intensity in Aerobics: Implications for Hearing Conservation." *Journal of the American Academy of Audiology* 14 (1):29–38.

Wright H. N., and R. Carhart. 1960. "The Efficiency of Binaural Listening among the Hearing Impaired." *Archives of Otolaryngology* 72:789–797.

Ylikoski, M. E. 1994. "Prolonged Exposure to Gunfire Noise among Professional Soldiers." *Scandinavian Journal of Work Environment and Health* 20 (2):87–92.

Zimmerman, A. 2004. "The Noisy Debate over Hearing Aids: Why So Expensive?" *Wall Street Journal,* March 24.

Index

acceptable noise level (ANL), 94–95
acceptance, of hearing loss, 93–94
acoustic neuroma, *see* acoustic tumor
acoustic tumor, 62, 126
activity level, 7
ADA (Americans with Disabilities
    Act), 108–109
aging, 7, 22–23, 27, 63, 86, 99, 133
air–bone gap, 39, 43
air conduction testing, 38, 39, 43–45
alarms, *see* alerting devices
alerting devices, 10, 102–104
Americans with Disabilities Act
    (ADA), 108–109
analog hearing aid, 72–77, 91–92
anger, 93
ANL (acceptable noise level), 94–95
antibiotics, 55
anvil, *see* incus
anxiety, 11, 13
artificial intelligence hearing aids, 120
assistive listening devices, 3, 64, 96,
    102–109, 149–150
associations, 139–142
audiogram, 40–46
audiologist, 2, 53–54, 82, 129–131,
    139–140
audiometric symbols, 40, 42
auricle, 29–31, 68
autoimmune inner ear disease, 60
avoidance, 14, 16

baby boomers: defined, 1, 18–21;
    shared experiences, 18–21, 26–27;
    special concerns, 21–27

baby bust, 2, 20
background noise, 11–12, 76, 84–85,
    90–92, 94–95, 98–100
BAHA, *see* bone-anchored hearing aid
barrel, talking in, *see* occlusion
    effect
Beethoven, Ludwig van, 59
behind-the-ear (BTE) hearing aid, 66,
    69–70, 82, 91
BICROS, *see* bilateral contralateral
    routing-of-signal hearing aid
bilateral contralateral routing-of-
    signal (BICROS) hearing aid, 71
body hearing aid, 70
bone-anchored hearing aid (BAHA),
    115–117, 145
bone conduction testing, 38–39,
    43–45
BTE, *see* behind-the-ear (BTE)
    hearing aid
buzzing, *see* feedback

cafeteria effect, 99
canal hearing aid, 66, 68, 82
caroverine, 112
central hearing loss, 36–37
cerumin, *see* earwax
cholesteatoma, 58
CIC, *see* completely-in-the-canal
    hearing aid
clinical audiologist, *see* audiologist
closed captioning, 107
cochlea, 30, 33
cochlear implant, 113–115, 121,
    143–145

cocktail party effect, *see* cafeteria effect
cognitive functioning, 11–12, 89
communication problems, *see* social functioning
completely-in-the-canal (CIC) hearing aid, 66–68, 72, 78, 82
concha hearing aid, *see* full-shell hearing aid
conductive hearing loss, 35–36, 39, 43–46, 58–59, 115–117
confidence, 10–11
contralateral routing-of-signal (CROS) hearing aid, 70–71, 116–117
CROS, *see* contralateral routing-of-signal hearing aid

decibel (dB), 41–42
denial, 7, 10, 16, 93–94, 136
dependency, 15–16, 85–86. *See also* independence
depression, 11, 13, 88–89
dexamethasone injection, 61
dexterity, 69, 78
diabetes, 51
digital feedback suppression, 118–120. *See also* feedback
digital hearing aid, 74–75, 91–92
disability, *see* handicap
disposable hearing aid, *see* noncustom-made hearing aid
distortion, 36, 72, 75–76, 85, 88
diuretics, 61
dizziness, 53, 60–62
doorbell, 102
drainage, 53, 55, 58

ear, anatomy, 28–34
ear canal, 29–31, 88
eardrum, 29–32, 55–58, 88; perforation, 35, 48, 56–58; repair, 56–57
ear hook, 66
ear impression, 82
earmold, 66, 69–70, 119, 125

earmuffs, 48–50, 136; amplified, 108; noise blocking, 48–50, 136
earplugs, 48–50, 136
earwax, 29, 34–36, 54, 57, 78–79
ebselen, 112
e-mail, 12, 106
employment, 2–3, 5–6, 12–13, 17, 25, 27
ENT physician, 54, 60, 126–128, 139–140
etidronate, 59
Eustachian tube, 30, 33, 55–56, 58
eyeglass hearing aid, 70
expectations, 7, 13, 16, 25–27, 63, 93
external otitis, 55

feedback, 77, 85–86, 118–120
firearms, 14, 49, 136
fluctuating hearing loss, 53, 60
FM system, 108–109
Food and Drug Administration (FDA), 126–132
frequency range of human ear, 40–41
frustration, 5, 12, 14–15
fullness in the ear, 48, 60, 62
full-shell hearing aid, 66, 69, 82

gamma knife radiosurgery, 62
gentamicin injection, 61

hair cells, *see* nerve cells
half-shell hearing aid, 68–68
hammer, *see* malleus
handicap, 7–9, 14, 17, 22–23, 37, 63
headphones, 107
head shadow effect, 71, 80. *See also* single-sided deafness
hearing aid: analyzer, 88; bands, 74–75; benefits, 64, 86–90, 95; channels, 74–75; circuits, 3, 72–75, 81, 91–92; comparison to other products, 90; complaints about, 84–86; cosmetic concerns, 67–70, 85–86; history, 65; landmarks, 66; manufacturers, 80–81; medical

examination requirement, 126–130; medical waiver, 126–130; multiple program, 72, 74–76, 90–92; noise reduction, 75; non-use, 3, 84–86; one versus two, 79–80; options, 68, 75–79, 81; performance, 71, 73–75, 88; prescriptive formulas, 72–73, 87–88; price, 71, 74, 81–83, 127, 130–132, 137; purchasing process, 82–83, 125–132; quality, 67, 81, 85, 91; removal cord, 66–68; satisfaction, 84–95; selecting, 80–81; styles, 65–71, 81, 90–91; trial, 82–83, 126; volume control, 72, 77–78, 92; wax guard, 78–79, 81; windscreen, 78, 81
hearing dogs, 103–104, 140
hearing instrument specialist, 82, 129–130
hearing loss: age-related, 1, 22–23, 36, 51, 63–64; causes, 34–35, 47–64; effect on others, 14–17; medically correctable, 35–36, 53–62; prevalence, 2, 21–23, 135–136; prevention, 47–53, 110–112, 134, 136–137; severity, 34, 42–43; types, 34–37; untreated, 13
Hearing Loss Association of America, *see* Self Help for Hard of Hearing People
hearing test, 37–46
hereditary hearing loss, 5, 34, 63–64
hertz (Hz), 41
high blood pressure, 50–51
high-frequency hearing loss, 48, 71, 102, 107

incus, 30–32
independence, 9–10, 88–89. *See also* dependence
idiopathic hearing loss, 64
infection, 34–35, 55–58, 126
inner ear, 33–34, 38–39, 48, 59, 61
insurance, 4, 95, 125, 133–134
Internet, 123–124

in-the-ear (ITE) hearing aid, *see* full-shell hearing aid
inverse square law, 97–98
isolation, 9, 11, 15, 88–89, 104
ITE (in-the-ear), *see* full-shell hearing aid

life expectancy, 1–2, 23
lifestyle, 2–4, 27, 67, 72, 75, 81
limitations, 2, 6–7, 16
linear amplification, 72–73. *See also* wide dynamic-range compression
lipreading, 99–100, 107, 114, 143
listening strategies, 96–101
localization of sound, 10, 79–80
loneliness, 9, 11, 13, 88–89
low-salt diet, 61

magnesium, 112
magnetic resonance imaging (MRI), 62
malleus, 30–32
masking, 42, 98
maximum power output (MPO), 73
Medicare, 133–134
Medline, 123
Ménière's disease, 60–61
microphone, 68, 76–77, 81, 92; directional, 68, 76–77, 81, 92, 118; omnidirectional, 76
middle ear, 29–33, 35, 39, 55–59
mild hearing loss, 3, 8–9, 36–37, 42–43, 67–69, 131
mini canal hearing aid, 66, 68
mixed hearing loss, 35–36, 44–46, 58–59
moderate hearing loss, 8, 43, 67–69, 131
moderately severe hearing loss, 43
mood, 6, 11, 13
MPO (maximum power output), 73
MRI (magnetic resonance imaging), 62
mumbling, 14
music, 14, 18–22, 36, 49
myringotomy, 55–56

National Institute on Deafness and
    Other Communication Disorders
    (NIDCD), 2, 21, 135, 141
National Institutes of Health (NIH),
    134–135, 141–142
nerve cell regeneration, 4, 122–123, 134
nerve cells, 33, 36, 48, 111–112, 114,
    122–123
nerve damage, *see* sensorineural
    hearing loss
neural response telemetry (NRT), 115
NIDCD, *see* National Institute on
    Deafness and Other Communica-
    tion Disorders
NIH, *see* National Institutes of Health
N-L-acetylcsteine, 112
noise exposure, 8, 14, 21–22, 34, 36,
    48–50, 52–53, 64, 112, 136–137
noncustom-made hearing aid, 71,
    130–132
normal hearing, 11, 40–44, 84–85,
    111–112
NRT (neural response telemetry), 115

OAEs (otoacoustic emissions),
    111–112
occlusion effect, 119–120
odor, 53, 58
open ear acoustics, 119–120
ossicles, 30–32, 35, 57–58
ossicular repair, 35, 57–58
otitis media, 55–56
otoacoustic emissions (OAEs), 111–112
otologist, *see* ENT physician
otorhinolaryngologist, *see* ENT
    physician
otosclerosis, 58–60, 110
ototoxicity, 51–53, 64
outer ear, 29–31, 35, 39, 55
oval window, 30–32
over-the-counter (OTC) hearing aids,
    130–132

pain, 22, 53, 55–56, 71
paranoia, 13

perforated eardrum, *see* eardrum:
    perforation
permanent threshold shift (PTS), 48
personal amplifier, 107–109, 130
Physicians' Desk Reference, 51
pinna, *see* auricle
presbycusis, 63–64. *See also* hearing
    loss: age-related
pressure equalization tube, 56
profound hearing loss, 43, 69–70,
    113–115
programmable hearing aid, 73–74, 91
PTS (permanent threshold shift), 48
publications, 142–144

quality-of-life, 2, 6–17, 27, 88–89,
    115, 137

radio, 99
real-ear hearing aid test, 88
relay service, *see* teletypewriter
remote control hearing aid, 78
repeating, 8, 15
research, on hearing, 4, 123–125,
    134–137
retirement, 2, 23–25, 27
reverberation, 5, 97, 99–100, 107
ringing in ears, *see* tinnitus
rock music, *see* music

safety, 3, 10, 80
security, 3, 10, 13
Self Help for Hard of Hearing People
    (SHHH), 142, 144
self-image, 6
semicircular canals, 30–31, 33–34
sensorineural hearing loss, 4, 35–36,
    39, 44–46, 50–51, 58–59, 62–64,
    85, 113–117
severe hearing loss, 9, 42–43, 46, 69,
    113, 131
SHHH (Self Help for Hard of Hearing
    People), 142, 144
signal-to-noise ratio, 99
sign language, 101, 109, 142

single-sided deafness, 80, 115–117
smoking, 50, 55
social functioning, 5–6, 8–9, 13,
    15–16, 93, 97
Social Security, 2, 133–134
sodium fluoride, 59–60
sound-level meter, 49
speech reception threshold (SRT),
    39, 43
speech recognition software, 120–121
SRT (speech reception threshold),
    39, 43
stapedectomy, 59–60, 110
stapes, 30–32, 59
steroid therapy, 60–62
stirrup, *see* stapes
stress, 11–12, 16–17
sudden hearing loss, 53, 61–62
swimmer's ear, 55
symptoms, red flag, 3, 53, 126, 128

TDD (telephone device for the deaf),
    see teletypewriter
telecoil, 65, 76–77, 81
telephone, 12, 65–67, 76–77, 104–106,
    121; amplified, 12, 105; answering
    machine, 106, 121; compatibility,
    3, 65, 67, 119; headset, 105
teletypewriter (TTY), 105–106
television, 14–15, 19, 98–99, 107
temporary threshold shift (TTS), 48–50

text messaging, 106
tinnitus, 5, 53, 62, 140
tiredness, 10–11
toxic medications, *see* ototoxicity
toxic substances, *see* ototoxicity
tragus, 68
TTS (temporary threshold shift),
    48–50
TTY (teletypewriter), 105–106
tympanic membrane, *see* eardrum
tympanoplasty, *see* eardrum: repair
trauma, 34, 48, 56–57
tubing, 66, 69–70

*United States v. National Society of
    Professional Engineers*, 129

vertigo, *see* dizziness
vestibular schwannoma, 62
vestibular system, 30, 33–34

Walsh-Healey Act, 48
WDRC, *see* wide dynamic-range
    compression
Western blot blood test, 60
wide dynamic-range compression
    (WDRC), 73–74, 87–88, 91–92
withdrawal, 16
word discrimination score testing,
    39–40, 43
work, *see* employment

About the Author

John M. Burkey is the director of audiology at the Lippy Group for Ear, Nose, and Throat in Warren, Ohio. He is author of *Overcoming Hearing Aid Fears: The Road to Better Hearing*, which was recognized by the *Library Journal* as one of the Best Consumer Health Books of 2003. He has also authored, coauthored, and contributed to articles published in hearing, hearing aid, and medical journals. Burkey is certified by the American Speech Language and Hearing Association and is a fellow of the American Academy of Audiology.